THE TRUTH ABOUT DRUGS

THE TRUTH ABOUT DRUGS

MARK J. KITTLESON, PH.D.
Southern Illinois University
General Editor

WILLIAM KANE, PH.D.
University of New Mexico
Adviser

RICHELLE RENNEGARBE, PH.D.
McKendree College
Adviser

Bruce Ragon
Principal Author

☑®

Facts On File, Inc.

The Truth About Drugs

Facts On File, Inc.
132 West 31st Street
New York NY 10001

Library of Congress Cataloging-in-Publication Data

The truth about drugs / Mark J. Kittleson, general editor; William Kane, adviser; Richelle Rennegarbe, adviser; Bruce Ragon, principal author.
    p. cm.
    Includes index
    ISBN 0-8160-5299-9 (hc: alk. paper)
    1. Drugs of abuse—Encyclopedias. 2. Drug abuse—Encyclopedias. I. Kittleson, Mark J., 1952– II. Ragon, Bruce
    RM316.T78 2004
    362.29—dc22   2004015217

Facts On File books are available at special discounts when purchased in bulk quantities for businesses, associations, institutions, or sales promotions. Please call our Special Sales Department in New York at (212) 967-8800 or (800) 322-8755.

You can find Facts On File on the World Wide Web at http://www.factsonfile.com.

Text design by David Strelecky
Cover design by Cathy Rincon
Graphs by Sholto Ainslie and Patricia Meschino

Printed in the United States of America

MP Hermitage 10 9 8 7 6 5 4 3 2 1

This book is printed on acid-free paper.

CONTENTS

LIST OF ILLUSTRATIONS AND TABLES

PREFACE

In developing The Truth About series, we have taken time to review some of the most pressing problems facing our youth today. Issues such as alcohol and drug abuse, depression, family problems, sexual activity, and eating disorders are at the top of a list of growing concerns. It is the intent of these books to provide vital facts while also dispelling myths about these terribly important and all-too-common situations. These are authoritative resources that kids can turn to in order to get an accurate answer to a specific question or to research the history of a problem, giving them access to the most current related data available. It is also a reference for parents, teachers, counselors, and others who work with youth and require detailed information.

Let's take a brief look at the issues associated with each of those topics. Alcohol and drug use and abuse continue to be a national concern. Today's young people often use drugs to avoid life's extraordinary pressures. In doing so they are losing their ability to learn how to cope effectively. Without the internal resources to cope with pressure, adolescents turn increasingly back to addictive behaviors. As a result, the problems and solutions are interrelated. Also, the speed with which the family structure is changing often leaves kids with no outlet for stress and no access to support mechanisms.

In addition, a world of youth faces the toughest years of their lives, dealing with the strong physiological urges that accompany sexual desire. Only when young people are presented the facts honestly, without indoctrination, are they likely to connect risk taking with certain behaviors. This reference set relies on knowledge as the most important tool in research and education.

Finally, one of the most puzzling issues of our times is that of eating disorders. Paradoxically, while our youth are obsessed with thinness and beauty and go to extremes to try to meet perceived societal expectations, they are also increasingly plagued by obesity. Here, too, separating the facts from fiction is an important tool in research and learning.

As much as possible, The Truth About presents the facts through honest discussions and reports of the most up-to-date research. Knowing the facts associated with health-related questions and problems will help young people make informed decisions in school and throughout life.

Mark J. Kittleson
General Editor

HOW TO
USE THIS BOOK

NOTE TO STUDENTS

Knowledge is power. By possessing knowledge you have the ability to make decisions, ask follow-up questions, or know where to go to obtain more information. In the world of health, that is power! That is the purpose of this book—to provide you the power you need to obtain unbiased, accurate information and *The Truth About Drugs*.

Topics in each volume of The Truth About are arranged in alphabetical order, from A to Z. Each of these entries defines its topic and explains in detail the particular issue. At the end of most entries are cross–references to related topics. A list of all topics by letter can be found in the table of contents or at the back of the book in the index.

How have these books been compiled? First, the publisher worked with me to identify some of the country's leading authorities on key issues in health education. These individuals were asked to identify some of the major concerns that young people have about such topics. The writers read the literature, spoke with health experts, and incorporated their own life and professional experiences to pull together the most up-to-date information on health issues, particularly those of interest to adolescents and of concern in *Healthy People 2010*.

Throughout the alphabetical entries, the reader will find sidebars that separate Fact from Fiction. There are Question-and-Answer boxes that attempt to address the most common questions that youth ask about sensitive topics. In addition, readers will find special features called "Teens Speak"—case studies of teens with personal stories related to the topic in hand.

This may be one of the most important books you will ever read. Please share it with your friends, families, teachers, and classmates. Remember, you possess the power to control your future. One way to affect your course is through the acquisition of knowledge. Good luck and keep healthy.

NOTE TO LIBRARIANS

This book, along with the rest of The Truth About series, serves as a wonderful resource for young researchers. It contains a variety of facts, case studies, and further readings that the reader can use to help answer questions, formulate new questions, or determine where to go to find more information. Even though the topics may be considered delicate by some, don't be afraid to ask patrons if they have questions. Feel free to direct them to the appropriate sources, but do not press them if you encounter reluctance. The best we can do as educators is to let young people know that we are there when they need us.

Mark J. Kittleson, Ph.D.
General Editor

ADDICTIVE BEHAVIORS AND DRUGS

Behaviors are considered addictive if one is unable to control them despite the fact that they produce significant negative physical or psychological effects. Drug addiction is the inability to stop using a drug despite negative physical or psychological effects. Addiction among teens is a topic of serious concern. Despite reductions in teen drug use in recent years, the 2003 "Monitoring the Future" study by the National Institute on Drug Abuse (NIDA) found that more than one-half of all 12th-grade students had used illegal drugs at least once. Almost one-quarter of 12th graders (24.1 percent) had used drugs in the 30 days prior to the survey.

RATES OF TEEN DRUG ABUSE

The "Monitoring the Future" study shows that substance abuse in the United States is a problem as early as eighth grade. According to the survey, 22.8 percent of eighth-grade students had tried illicit drugs, and 9.7 percent had used drugs in the previous 30 days. The study also found abuse of substances other than illegal drugs. Over three-quarters of all 12th graders reported having used alcohol at least once, and 47.5 percent had used it in the previous 30 days. Among eighth graders, 45.6 percent had used alcohol at least once, and 19.7 percent admitted to using it within 30 days of the survey. Over one-half (53.7 percent) of 12th graders had tried cigarettes, as had 28.4 percent of eighth graders.

The Youth Risk Behavior Surveillance System, a national survey of teen drug behaviors completed by the Centers for Disease Control and Prevention (CDC) in 2001, showed that within 30 days preceding the survey, almost 31 percent of students rode in a car with a driver who

1

had consumed alcohol and over 13 percent had driven a car while under the influence of alcohol. The survey also reported that almost 29 percent of students had been offered, sold, or given an illegal drug on school property within the last 12 months. Among the students surveyed, 2.3 percent had injected an illegal drug, 5 percent had used anabolic steroids (drugs used the increase strength and muscle mass), over 9 percent had used **cocaine** (a highly addictive stimulant drug derived from the coca plant), almost 10 percent had used **methamphetamines** (drugs that stimulate the nervous system), and roughly 15 percent had used inhalants (sniffed glue, breathed aerosols, or inhaled paints). These statistics reveal that peer pressure to engage in drug use would most likely involve an inhalant, methamphetamine, or cocaine.

COMMONLY ABUSED DRUGS

Although statistics vary, **marijuana** remains the most used illicit drug among teens. The CDC reported in a nationwide study conducted in 2001 that roughly 42 percent of students in grades nine through 12 had tried marijuana. The rate of teen marijuana use is almost three times greater than that of the second most frequently used drugs (inhalants, used by 15 percent of students). **Marijuana** use is four times greater than the use of methamphetamines (10 percent of students) and cocaine (9 percent), the third and fourth most frequently used drugs. The use of **sedatives**, **designer drugs**, steroids, and **opiates** is less widespread among teens.

A category of drugs called **club drugs** has become increasingly popular among teens because of drug use at "raves," parties, and dance clubs. Club drugs typically include MDMA (ecstasy), gamma-hydroxybutyrate (GHB), Rohypnol (roofies), and ketamine. According to www.clubdrugs.org, an online service of NIDA, these drugs may cause serious health problems. They can be even more dangerous if taken in combination with alcohol. Some club drugs have been identified as "date rape drugs" or "predatory drugs." These drugs can knock out a person and cause him or her to forget what happened for some time afterward. Because of this effect, these drugs have been used to render people unconscious and make them vulnerable to sexual assault. The federal government has recently passed several new laws to help protect victims of these easily disguised drugs.

CAUSES OF DRUG ABUSE

Researchers disagree about the causes of drug abuse. Some suggest that a tendency to engage in addictive behavior is hereditary. Others believe that factors in a person's environment, or surroundings, may contribute to drug abuse. It seems likely that some combination of biological and environmental factors causes drug abuse. However, social scientists have closely studied several potential causes of drug abuse, including **social skills,** psychological health, and the family.

Research has found that teens with poor **social skills**—those who have not succeeded in establishing good relations with others of their own age—are more likely than other teenagers to abuse drugs. So are those who show inappropriate social behaviors such as sudden and unprovoked violence toward others. Teens with poor social skills often seek support and friendship from one another. Gangs often offer the kind of acceptance that these troubled teens do not find elsewhere. Gang members may reinforce each other's inappropriate behaviors, including drug use.

Serious emotional and psychological problems are also related to drug abuse. A 1999 Substance Abuse and Mental Health Services Administration (SAMHSA) study titled "The Relationship Between Mental Health and Substance Abuse Among Adolescents" found that teens with serious psychological problems were seven times more likely to abuse drugs or alcohol than teens with few or no emotional problems. Psychologically troubled teens were nearly nine times as likely to require treatment for drug abuse.

According to a 2001 SAMHSA study titled "Parental Influences on Adolescent Marijuana Use and the Baby Boom Generation," parents exert significant influence on teen drug use. The study reported that teens whose parents displayed antidrug attitudes were less likely to use drugs than teens whose parents were neutral or approving of drug use. Interestingly, teens with parents who expressed antidrug sentiments were less likely to use drugs even if they knew their parents had at one time experimented with drugs.

Other family characteristics are related to drug use as well. SAMHSA's 2002 National Survey on Drug Use and Health (formerly called the National Household Survey on Drug Abuse) found that drug abuse is less likely among families with higher levels of income and education. Where one lives also impacts the likelihood of drug use. Teens in cities are more likely to abuse drugs than those in small towns or rural areas.

EFFECTS OF DRUG ABUSE

Drug abuse has profound effects not only on the user but also the user's family, friends, community, and workplace. Drug abuse is associated with a wide variety of negative consequences such as shattered families, gang activity, neighborhood decay, and crime. Law enforcement agencies spend billions of dollars per year combating drugs and drug-related crime, and thousands of people are sentenced to prison each year for drug offenses.

Scientists have noted many adverse physical and psychological effects of drugs, which vary from one drug to another. For example, marijuana can cause problems with memory and learning, distorted perception, difficulty in thinking and problem solving, and loss of coordination. Long-term complications can include lung damage and suppression of the immune system. Other drugs can cause even more serious problems. Cocaine, amphetamines, and heroin can produce psychological symptoms including **paranoia**, **hallucinations**, and **delusions** and physical problems such as increased heart rate, convulsions, coma, and even death. Taking a dangerous overdose (an amount high enough to cause an adverse reaction) is also a possibility with most drugs.

Historically, drug and alcohol abuse can also lead to severe family disruption. According to a 1991 study, "Psychiatric Disorders in America: The Epidemiologic Catchment Area Study," 24.2 percent of all Americans who had been divorced or separated more than once were alcoholics. Fewer than 9 percent of those in intact marriages were alcoholics. A 1991 article titled "Homeless and Dual Diagnosis" reported that 30–40 percent of the nation's homeless have a substance abuse problem. In addition, the U.S. Conference of Mayors found that domestic violence was a primary cause of homelessness. This is significant because 80 percent of 915 child-welfare professionals surveyed in 1997 by the National Center of Addiction and Substance Abuse at Columbia University said that substance abuse directly causes or plays a role in most cases of child abuse.

Several studies demonstrate the negative impact of drug abuse on communities. A 1990 study titled "Drug Marketing, Property Crime, and Neighborhood Viability: Organized Crime Connections," reported that drug sales lead to increasing crime and violence. According to the 2002 National Crime Victimization Survey, 29 percent of victims of violent crime reported that the offender was using drugs or alcohol at the time of the crime. More affluent residents move out, leaving those with fewer resources to deal with the problem. Increases in violent crimes such as assaults and murder and property crimes such as burglary and theft cause property values to fall, which in turn may lead to community decay.

Drugs also impact the productivity and profitability of businesses. The 1997 National Household Survey on Drug Abuse reported that 7.7 percent of all American workers used alcohol or drugs at the workplace. Alcohol, marijuana, and cocaine are the drugs most frequently abused in the workplace. According to SAMHSA, alcoholics and problem drinkers are four to eight times more likely to be absent for work than sober workers. Those who abuse other substances miss an average of five days of work per month and are 33 percent less productive than sober workers. In 1995, productivity losses attributed to alcohol abuse in the workplace reached $119 billion. That figure does not include losses due to the use of other drugs.

Despite the widespread negative effects of drug and alcohol abuse, many teens do not take the issue seriously enough. Some mistakenly think that drugs are not as harmful as they have been led to believe. Others are convinced that they can easily resist the temptation to use drugs. Such assumptions can be dangerously mistaken. Many teens have no intention of doing drugs but may end up experimenting because of curiosity or peer pressure. Once a teen starts using drugs, he or she may find it difficult to stop. This book attempts to give you the information you need about the dangers of drug abuse and help you make the wise choice to avoid using drugs.

RISKY BUSINESS SELF-TEST

The following test is designed to let you find out more about your own risk of abusing drugs. Record you answers on a sheet of paper.

Are you at risk of abusing drugs?

Answer "true" or "false" to these questions to assess whether you may be at risk of abusing drugs or alcohol.

- Many of my friends use drugs.
- I use drugs to help me get through the day.
- I can stop using drugs at any time.
- I smoke and drink regularly.
- Marijuana is no big deal.
- Drugs do not affect my health.

- I have little interest in school and my grades show it.
- I argue with my parents a lot.
- I am often influenced by my peers to smoke or drink.
- Drugs are available at my school.
- I go to raves or dance parties regularly.
- Club drugs are fun to take and have no long-term consequences.
- Several of my friends have been arrested at least once.
- Some of my friends sell drugs.
- I belong to a gang or am friends with gang members.
- I have been taking pills to control my weight for over a year.
- Parties I attend usually have drugs and alcohol available.
- I pass out due to drugs and/or alcohol at least once a month.
- I don't do drugs; I only get drunk and smoke.

If you answered "true" to one or more of these statements, you may be at an increased risk for drug abuse or are already on your way to being addicted. Alcohol abuse and smoking have been shown to lead to drug use. Having friends that use drugs and having positive attitudes toward drugs also indicate a strong possibility of future drug use.

Peer pressure is a very powerful force and attending parties or being in other situations where peer influence to use drugs is strong can lead to drug use. Denial of drug abuse or addiction is a major stumbling block to seeking help. Realizing that you can no longer control your drug use is critical to the recovery process.

See also: Dependence and Addiction; Depression and Drugs; Drug Abuse, Causes of; Gangs and Drugs; Inhalants; Injection Drugs; Overdose and Drugs; Peer Pressure and Drugs; Risk Factors and Risk Taking; Steroids, Anabolic

A TO Z ENTRIES

■ ADDICTION AND DEPENDENCE
See: Dependence and Addiction

■ ALCOHOL AND ALCOHOL ABUSE
See: Drugs and Drinking

■ CLUB AND DESIGNER DRUGS
Synthetically produced substances from a variety of drug categories that have a range of effects from increasing alertness to dulling pain. The name "club drugs" comes from the fact that these drugs first gained popularity among young people who used them at dance clubs to heighten their sensory experiences. They are also called "designer drugs," because they are not naturally occurring substances but created, or designed, in underground laboratories. Because there is little quality control in the production of these drugs, it is difficult to know exactly what chemicals are used to make them and in what dosages. That means it can be difficult to predict what effect they will have from one usage to the next. This is one of the factors that makes club drugs so dangerous.

The most commonly used club drugs are ecstasy (MDMA), GHB (gamma-hydroxybutyrate), roofies (Rohypnol), and Special K (ketamine). Some of these drugs act as **stimulants**, increasing the user's alertness and decreasing fatigue. Others are **depressants** that cause drowsiness and impair motor coordination. Still others produce effects similar to **hallucinogens**. When mixed, these widely varying types of drug actions can have serious negative consequences.

ECSTASY
Ecstasy, or MDMA (3–4 methylenedioxy-methamphetamine), is the most popular club or designer drug. It is a synthetic drug that is chemically similar to the stimulant **methamphetamine** and the hallucinogen **mescaline**. It goes by a variety of names, including Adam, XTC, hug, beans, and love drug. The effects of ecstasy include increased alertness and energy sometimes accompanied by **euphoria** (a feeling of elation) and **hallucinations** (distorted perceptions). Ecstasy has also

gained popularity because of its reputation for heightening sexual pleasure and reducing the user's sensitivity to pain.

Users of ecstasy face many of the same risks as those who use other stimulants. These include increases in heart rate and blood pressure, muscle tension, involuntary teeth clenching, nausea, blurred vision, faintness, and chills or sweating. In high doses, ecstasy can interfere with the body's ability to regulate temperature. This can cause a sharp increase in body temperature known as hyperthermia, which can lead to liver, kidney, and cardiovascular system failure. Ecstasy can interfere with the body's ability to break down the drug. As a result, potentially harmful levels of the drug can accumulate inside a user's body with repeated doses over a short period of time. On rare occasions, an overdose of ecstasy can be fatal.

Ecstasy works by affecting nerve cells in the brain that use the chemical serotonin to communicate with other nerve cells. Long-term use can disrupt the serotonin system, which plays an important role in regulating mood, aggression, sexual activity, sleep, and sensitivity to pain. Research in animals indicates that ecstasy may actually kill nerve cells in the brain. Scientists are currently researching the drug to see if it has the same effects on humans.

According to the National Institute on Drug Abuse (NIDA), chronic (long-term) ecstasy users may experience both cognitive and psychological disorders. Ecstasy users perform more poorly than nonusers on certain cognitive or memory tasks. However, some of these effects may be due to the use of other drugs in combination with MDMA. Psychological effects of use can include confusion, depression, sleep problems, drug cravings, and severe anxiety. These problems can occur during and sometimes days or weeks after taking ecstasy. Research in animals suggests that chronic use can damage neurons that are involved in mood, thinking, and judgment.

NIDA warns that other drugs chemically similar to MDMA are sometimes sold as ecstasy. These drugs can create additional health risks to the user. Also, drugs sold as ecstasy may contain other substances in addition to MDMA, such as the stimulant ephedrine, the cough suppressant dextromethorphan, another club drug called ketamine, caffeine, **cocaine**, and methamphetamine. The combination of ecstasy with one or more of these drugs can be very dangerous, especially if the user also consumes substances such as **marijuana** and alcohol when taking ecstasy.

According to the National Survey on Drug Use and Health conducted by the Substance Abuse and Mental Health Services Administration (SAMHSA), an estimated 676,000 people in the United States age 12 and older used ecstasy in 2002. The University of Michigan's 2003 "Monitoring the Future" study reported a recent decline in the use of ecstasy among teens. According to the study, 2.9 percent of eighth graders used ecstasy in 2002 compared with 2.1 percent in 2003. Use among 10th graders declined from 4.9 percent to 3.0 percent, and ecstasy use dropped from 7.4 percent to 4.5 percent among 12th graders. These numbers are encouraging, as they indicate that young people are growing more aware of the dangers of ecstasy.

GHB

Gamma-hydroxybutyrate, or GHB, is a central nervous system depressant that was widely available as an **over-the-counter drug** in health-food stores until 1992. According to NIDA, GHB abuse in the United States began around 1990. Bodybuilders frequently purchased GHB to quickly reduce fat and build muscles. Other users began taking it for its **sedative** effects and its ability to produce a state of euphoria. Street names for GHB include liquid ecstasy, soap, easy lay, vita-G, and Georgia home boy.

At lower doses, GHB produces a euphoria similar to alcohol, generating the feeling of being relaxed, happy, and sociable. At higher doses, dizziness, vomiting, and muscle spasms can occur. Other symptoms of GHB use include lethargy (sluggishness), extreme intoxication, impaired judgment, nausea, vomiting, and dizziness. The drug can also cause unconsciousness, depression, seizures, severe respiratory depression, and coma. Symptoms appear within 15–20 minutes of taking the drug and can last between two and three hours but may linger for an entire day. Mixing GHB with alcohol is extremely dangerous, because both drugs depress the central nervous system. Combining GHB and alcohol has resulted in a number of deaths, typically from respiratory failure.

The 2003 "Monitoring the Future" study showed that use of GHB by high school students remained about the same between 2002 and 2003. In 2003, use of GHB among eighth graders was 0.9 percent, use among 10th graders was 1.4 percent, and 1.4 percent of 12th graders reported using GHB in the previous year.

Fact Or Fiction?

The use of designer drugs can cause brain damage.

Fact: According to a 1995 article in the *Journal of Neuroscience* titled "Reorganization of Ascending 5-HT Axon Projections in Animals Previously Exposed to the Recreational Drug 3,4-methelene-dioxymethamphetamine (MDMA, ecstasy)," even a single dose of ecstasy may significantly damage brain cells. In the study, researchers found that monkeys who had been given ecstasy showed damage to certain nerve cells that later grew back abnormally or not at all. Researchers are working to determine if these findings also apply to human beings exposed to ecstasy. Dr. George Ricuarte, who conducted the study, is currently doing new research using brain-imaging techniques to evaluate the possibility of long-term brain damage in humans who have previously used either methamphetamine or ecstasy.

ROHYPNOL

Rohypnol is the brand name for a commercially produced drug called flunitrazepam. It belongs to the class of drugs known as benzodiazepines—antianxiety drugs that include Librium and Valium. Rohypnol is not approved for use in the United States and cannot be legally imported from other countries. Rohypnol began to appear in the United States in the early 1990s, shortly after GHB became popular as a club drug. Common names for Rohypnol include rophies, roofies, roach, and rope.

The effects of Rohypnol include muscle relaxation and slowed motor responses. Rohypnol also decreases blood pressure, causes the body to retain urine, and produces an intoxicated feeling similar to that of alcohol. The most serious effect produced by Rohypnol is anterograde amnesia—the inability to remember events that take place after the drug is taken. Rohypnol may be lethal when mixed with alcohol and/or other depressants. The 2003 "Monitoring the Future" study found that 0.5 percent of eighth graders, 0.6 percent of 10th graders, and 1.3 percent of 12th graders reported using Rohypnol in the past year.

KETAMINE

Originally created as an anesthetic around 1970, ketamine is widely used in both human and animal medicine. About 90 percent of the ketamine sold legally in the United States is used in veterinary practice. However, ketamine is also abused because of its ability to produce euphoria, dreamlike states, and hallucinations. In high doses, ketamine can cause confusion, amnesia, impaired motor function, high blood pressure, depression, and potentially fatal respiratory problems. Ketamine is also known as Special K or vitamin K.

TEENS SPEAK

A lot of kids seem to be trying club drugs these days, but after what happened to my friend the other day, I'm not going to be one of them.

My friends and I really love to dance, and we go to clubs on the weekends. We don't go to drink or do drugs, we just like hanging out, dancing, listening to the music, and talking. A few weeks ago, I made friends with a new girl in school named Kim. She was really cool and was also into dancing, so I invited her to come with us to the clubs that weekend.

When Kim met my friends on Friday night, everyone hit it off with her. She seemed sure of herself but not cocky or anything like that. After we'd been at the club for about 15 minutes, Kim went to the bathroom. A few minutes after she came out, I noticed she looked kind of strange. Her eyes were sort of glassy, and she seemed to be super pumped-up. For the next hour or so she was all over the dance floor—I'd never seen anybody who had so much energy.

After about an hour or so, however, Kim started acting really weird. She was really thirsty and her whole body was flushed. She started shaking and feeling weak and sick to her stomach. We were all really scared because she looked terrible and was acting so sick. We got her outside and sat her down, and then one of my friends called 911. Before the ambulance got there, Kim told me she had taken some ecstasy when she went to the bathroom. At first it made her feel great, like she had all the energy in the world. Then she suddenly started feeling like she was going to die. Thankfully the emergency technicians in the ambulance were able to get her feeling better, but they took her to the emergency room just to be sure she was OK.

Kim taught me a big lesson. You don't need drugs to have a good time, and in fact they will ruin the good times you have. Kim is fine now, but I don't think she'll be doing ecstasy again.

CLUB DRUGS AND DATE RAPE

In recent years, health and law enforcement officials have become concerned about the use of club drugs known as **date rape drugs** (substances used to render a person unconscious and susceptible to date rape). Rohypnol, GHB, and ketamine are commonly identified as date rape drugs. When slipped into a drink, these drugs can not only cause unconsciousness but also leave the victim with no memory of what happened.

If someone you know appears to be dizzy, confused, or suffering from other sudden, unexplained symptoms after having a drink, they may have been drugged. If you suspect that you or someone you know has been drugged, find medical help immediately. Rohypnol, GHB, and alcohol all depress the functioning of the central nervous system. Combining these drugs with alcohol can slow the user's heart rate and breathing to dangerously low levels. The combination can result in coma or even death from respiratory failure.

According to NIDA, teen use of club and designer drugs increased dramatically during the 1990s, reaching a peak around 2000. The numbers began to decline thereafter, but the percentage of teens using ecstasy in 2003 was still three times as high as it was just seven years earlier. Although progress is clearly being made in alerting teens to the dangers of club drugs, many are still taking serious risks by using these substances.

See also: Drugs and Drinking; Illegal Drugs, Common; Overdose and Drugs; Sexual Behavior and Drug Abuse

FURTHER READING
Balkin, Karen F. and Louise Gerdes. *Club Drugs.* Portland, OR: Greenhaven Press, 2004.
Brennan, Kristine. *Ecstasy and Other Designer Drugs.* London, UK: Chelsea House Publications, 1999.

Knowles, Cynthia R. *Up All Night: A Closer Look at Club Drugs and Rave Culture.* Thousand Oaks, CA: Red House Press, 2001.

Robbins, Paul R. *Designer Drugs.* London, UK: Enslow Publishers, 1995.

■ CRACK COCAINE

A concentrated and more addictive form of **cocaine,** an illegal drug derived from the coca plant. Crack cocaine produces more profound effects than other forms of the drug. Both cocaine and crack cocaine are **stimulants,** substances that tend to increase alertness, energy, and physical activity. Although cocaine has been used for more than 100 years, crack is a relatively new drug that first appeared in the United States in the early 1980s. Since that time, its use has grown rapidly, and law enforcement officials consider it among the most dangerous of illegal drugs.

DESCRIPTION AND EFFECTS

Cocaine is a white powder produced by chemically treating the leaves of the coca plant. Coca leaves contain a natural stimulant whose effects are greatly increased as a result of chemical treatment. Crack is produced by dissolving powdered cocaine in a mixture of water and ammonia or sodium bicarbonate (baking soda). The mixture is boiled until a solid substance forms. The solid is then removed from the liquid, dried, and broken into chunks (known as "rocks") that are sold as crack cocaine. The most common methods of administering powder cocaine are by snorting (inhaling through the nose) and through intravenous injection. By contrast, crack cocaine is usually smoked in a pipe. The smoke carries the drug into the user's lungs where it is absorbed quickly into the bloodstream. Crack gets its name from the cracking sound the drug makes when it is heated.

The short-term effects of crack are similar to those of cocaine and include **euphoria,** stimulation of the **central nervous system** (the brain and the spinal cord), reduced fatigue, and a sense of mental clarity. Because crack is smoked, it is absorbed more quickly into the body and produces a more intense reaction than snorting powder cocaine. However, the faster the drug is absorbed, the shorter the duration of its effect. The short-term effects of crack typically last only about 5–10 minutes. Frequent use of crack can lead to **tolerance** of the drug, a condition in which the user must increase his or her intake of the drug to achieve the same effects. At higher doses crack use can lead to **paranoia** and trigger aggressive behavior. Long-term effects include restlessness, irritability, and anxiety.

Crack also produces physical effects similar to those of cocaine, including increased temperature, elevated heart rate and blood pressure, constriction (narrowing) of blood vessels, loss of appetite, convulsions, muscle twitching, and irregular heartbeat. In rare instances, sudden death may occur directly as a result of use. According to the National Institute on Drug Abuse, crack-related deaths are often a result of heart attack or seizure followed by respiratory system failure.

Statistics on medical emergency calls related to crack indicate just how serious the effects of the drug can be. In 2002, emergency rooms and emergency medical personnel across the United States reported 42,146 crack "mentions" to the Drug Abuse Warning Network (DAWN), a nationwide clearinghouse for information on drug use. A "mention" refers to a report made by the emergency patient or a third party that the patient used a particular drug prior to the emergency episode. More than one out of five cocaine mentions (21 percent of the total) during 2002 concerned crack cocaine. Despite the large number of crack mentions for 2002, the figure actually represents a decline from the previous year's total of 46,964.

Q & A

Question: What is a crack baby?

Answer: A crack baby is an infant that experiences physical and behavioral problems as a result of the use of crack by his or her mother during pregnancy. A 1996 article titled "Maternal Exposure to Crack Cocaine Produces Stressed Newborns" (Brown University News Bureau) reported that babies exposed to crack while in the womb showed abnormal patterns of both excitability and lethargy (sluggishness) compared with nonexposed infants. In addition, babies exposed to crack appeared more stressed. They often were unable to follow certain stimuli such as a rattle or bell compared with nonexposed infants. According to the article, crack babies "were more jittery, had more muscle tension, and were harder to move because they were stiff." Some were also drowsier and had a weaker crawl than nonexposed babies.

Some experts dispute the idea that crack is responsible for these developmental difficulties. A 2001 report by the *Journal of the*

American Medical Association suggested that most of the problems experienced by these infants were related to other risk factors such as cigarettes, alcohol, and poverty. The research found no consistent link between crack exposure before birth and childhood physical growth or development. The researchers did discover that motor skill problems linked to crack exposure typically disappeared by the time the child was seven months old. However, the report also concluded that more research was needed on the drug's effects on an infant's nervous system. One of the authors of the report remarked, "Although it would be inaccurate to say that we're absolutely sure that there are no adverse physical or mental effects of prenatal cocaine exposure, I think we can say that the popular stereotype of the distraught child who is unable to love and unable to learn is absolutely inaccurate."

INCIDENCE OF USE

A number of government- and university-sponsored studies indicate that crack cocaine use is a serious problem in the United States. The Substance Abuse and Mental Health Services Administration (SAMHSA), a division of the Department of Health and Human Services, compiles an annual report on drug use titled the "National Survey on Drug Use and Health." According to SAMHSA's 2002 findings, 8.4 million Americans age 12 and older reported trying crack at least once. This figure represents 3.6 percent of the population age 12 or older. Some 567,000 of those who smoked crack in 2002 reported using it in the month prior to the survey.

The University of Michigan's 2003 "Monitoring the Future" study, which tracked drug use among eighth-, 10th-, and 12th-grade students, suggests that crack use is a problem among teens. However, the study also found that teen crack use has declined slightly in recent years. According to the study, in 2002 some 2.5 percent of eighth graders, 3.6 percent of 10th graders, and 3.8 percent of 12th graders reported using crack cocaine at least once. The figures for eighth graders remained unchanged in 2003, but the study found that crack use declined to 2.7 percent among 10th graders and 3.6 percent among 12th graders. The 2003 study also reported that 1.6 percent of eighth and 10th graders and 2.2 percent of 12th graders had smoked crack in the previous year.

Students who responded to the 2003 "Monitoring the Future" study reported that they had little difficulty in obtaining crack cocaine. A significant percentage of students from all three grades also reported that they did not consider using crack once or twice to be extremely risky behavior. According to the study, 22.5 percent of eighth graders, 29.6 percent of 10th graders, and 35.3 percent of 12th graders surveyed in 2003 said that crack cocaine was "fairly easy" or "very easy" to obtain. The study found that fewer than half of eighth graders (48.7 percent) and 12th graders (47.3 percent) agreed with the statement that trying crack once or twice represented a "great risk." Over half of 10th graders (57.6 percent) agreed that using crack even once was a "great risk."

Crack is also strongly linked to criminal behavior. According to the National Institute of Justice's Arrestee Drug Abuse Monitoring Program (ADAM), 17.2 percent of adult males arrested for criminal offenses in 2002 and 24.5 percent of adult female arrestees reported using crack cocaine at least once in the year before being arrested. In 2002, the Drug Enforcement Administration (DEA) made 5,166 arrests involving crack cocaine, which represented 20.2 percent of all drug arrests for the year.

TEENS SPEAK

My name is Erin, and I want to warn you about a drug that many kids don't think is a serious problem: crack. I live in a middle-class neighborhood and go to a good school. I always though of crack as something that was only found in the poorest parts of the inner city. I never imagined that kids in the suburbs were doing it, especially kids that I knew. I found out differently a few weeks ago.

Jim is a guy in many of my classes. He's not really a close friend, more of an acquaintance. I knew he liked to party; I've seen him drinking beer and smoking weed a couple of times. I also heard that he did some harder drugs like cocaine, but I never believed those stories. He seemed like a pretty level-headed guy and never struck me as someone who would risk messing himself up with cocaine.

Then one week I noticed that I hadn't seen Jim around school for several days. I asked a friend who also knew Jim if she had any idea where he was. She told me she had heard that he was in the hospital. When I asked what was wrong with him, she said he had a heart attack. I was shocked. Jim is only 16, and he is in good shape—he is even on the basketball team. How in the world did someone like that suffer a heart attack? My friend said it happened after Jim smoked crack. Someone who was there told her that Jim collapsed after smoking a single "rock" of crack. The other kids were really freaked out, but they called 911, and the emergency crew was able to get Jim to the hospital in time to save his life.

My friend said the kids with Jim were all scared to death, and they have all sworn off smoking crack again. Unfortunately it was too late for Jim. I hear he's going to recover, but he'll never be the same, and I'll never again think of crack as someone else's problem.

THE CRACK EPIDEMIC

According to the DEA, an oversupply of powder cocaine in the Bahamas in the early 1980s led to the introduction of crack in the United States. At that time most of the cocaine shipped to the United States came through the Bahamas, and by 1980 the price on the islands had dropped by as much as 80 percent as a result of an over-supply. Dealers there needed to find a way to convert the powder into a form that was cheap, easy to produce, ready to use, and profitable. The result was crack, and by 1981 the drug was appearing in Los Angeles, San Diego, and Houston. Later, Caribbean immigrants taught dealers in Miami how to produce crack, and before long the drug had spread throughout the United States.

Crack cocaine had advantages for both the user and the dealer. It was not only purer than powder cocaine (which often contains other substances to increase the volume) but also cheaper. It also produced an instant and much stronger "high" than powder cocaine. For the user, this new form of cocaine meant a more intense experience; for the dealer, it meant that users became addicted more quickly, resulting in increased demand. Users needed to smoke more and more frequently to achieve the same effects.

At first, law enforcement officials did not consider crack to be a serious problem, mainly because it was popular primarily among middle-class users rather than cocaine addicts. In fact, many were convinced that crack use was confined largely to Miami until it appeared in New York City in December 1983. As in Miami, crack in New York was largely a middle-class drug at first. The DEA estimated that more than 75 percent of early crack users in New York were white professionals, middle-class teens from Long Island and New Jersey, or users from upper-class Westchester County. However, because of its extremely low price, crack soon spread to lower-class and poor neighborhoods. By early 1986, crack was firmly entrenched in the inner city and by the end of the year had spread to 28 states and the District of Columbia. By 1987, crack was available in all but four states and by the following year it had replaced heroin as the biggest drug problem in Detroit.

The crack epidemic had two serious negative social effects: it substantially increased the number of cocaine addicts in the United States and it led to a wave of drug-related violence. According to SAMHSA's National Household Survey on Drug Abuse, the number of people who admitted using cocaine on a routine basis increased from 4.2 million in 1984 to 5.8 million in 1985. DAWN reported that cocaine-related hospital emergencies increased by 12 percent from 1984 to 1985 and by 110 percent between 1985 and 1986. Between 1984 and 1987, the number of cocaine-related emergency incidents increased some 400 percent.

As selling crack became more profitable, both the number of traffickers and the violence associated with its sale increased. By the late 1980s, the DEA reported that more than 10,000 gang members were dealing drugs in the United States and that crack was a significant source of their income. According to a 1988 study by the Bureau of Justice Statistics, crack use was related to 32 percent of all homicides and 60 percent of drug-related homicides in New York City. On a nearly daily basis, the news broadcasters reported drive-by shootings related to crack dealing.

Fact Or Fiction?

The Central intelligence Agency (CIA) is responsible for bringing crack cocaine to the United States.

Fact: A series of news reports published in the *San Jose Mercury* newspaper in 1995 claimed that during the 1980s rebels attempting to overthrow the Nicaraguan government were introducing massive amounts of crack cocaine into the United States with the approval and even support of the CIA. According to Gary Webb, author of the articles, profits from crack sales funded the revolution being carried out by the rebels, known as the contras. The U.S. government has strongly disputed Webb's claims, but Webb stands by his story, which was told to him by drug dealers heavily involved in the San Francisco-area crack trade in the 1980s. Webb later published a book titled *Dark Alliance: The CIA, the contras, and the Crack Cocaine Explosion*, which laid out his case against the CIA.

LAW ENFORCEMENT RESPONSES TO CRACK

By 1986, the crack problem in the United States had become so serious that Congress passed the Anti-Drug Abuse Act, which included $8 million to help law enforcement combat domestic cocaine trafficking. The bill also called for $1.5 million in funding to establish crack task forces in Los Angeles, Houston, Minneapolis, Denver, and Detroit. At the same time, the DEA embarked on a program to reduce the amount of cocaine entering the country by attacking major international drug trafficking rings. By the late 1980s, the DEA, the Department of Justice, and state and local law enforcement agencies all boasted crack task forces. Cocaine became the main focus of the DEA's activities, and cocaine arrests accounted for nearly 65 percent of the DEA's total arrests in 1988.

One of the more controversial features of the Anti-Drug Abuse Act of 1986 was that it created a legal distinction between "cocaine base" (crack and the liquid mixture from which crack is created) and other forms of cocaine. The act also introduced mandatory minimum penalties for federal drug trafficking offenses that were based on the type and quantity of drug sold. Together, these developments resulted in harsher penalties for selling crack than for other drug offenses. Under the law, a defendant convicted of dealing 1.75 ounces, or 50 grams, of crack would receive the same sentence as someone who sold 100-times as much (11 pounds, or five kilograms) powder cocaine. According to a 1995 report by the U.S. Sentencing Commission, crack is the only drug for which a first-time offender can receive a mandatory minimum sentence.

In the 1990s, the federal sentencing guidelines concerning crack were under attack by those who claimed the law was racially discriminatory. These claims stemmed from research that showed that, following passage of the law, black drug offenders were much more likely to receive tougher sentences than white offenders. According to a 1992 Federal Judicial Center report, "The General Effect of Mandatory Prison Terms: A Longitudinal Study of Federal Sentences Imposed," the difference in the average sentences for blacks and whites convicted of drug offenses increased dramatically after passage of the 1986 act. Prior to 1986, black offenders convicted of federal drug offenses received sentences that averaged 11 percent longer than those given to white offenders. By 1990, the average sentence for black drug offenders was 49 percent higher than those for whites. The perception among many observers was that crack offenders were being punished more harshly than powder cocaine offenders, because crack was associated in the public mind with lower-class blacks while powder cocaine was seen as a drug used by middle-class whites.

In a special report to Congress in 1997, the U.S. Sentencing Commission agreed with many of the race-based criticisms of the 1986 act. For example, the commission found that although the majority of crack users were white, nearly 90 percent of convicted crack dealers were black. The commission concluded that "sentences appear to be harsher and more severe for racial minorities than others as a result of this law." The commission also noted problems with the way law enforcement officials investigated and prosecuted cases involving crack. The commission was concerned that even when law enforcement agencies were aware that a suspect possessed powder cocaine, they may wait to arrest the suspect until he or she had converted it into crack because of the stiffer sentences given to convicted crack dealers. The report suggested that such law enforcement practices seemed more likely to occur when the suspect was African American.

The 1997 U.S. Sentencing Commission report also found that convicted crack dealers received average sentences as harsh or harsher than those for many violent crimes. Defendants convicted for crack offenses under the 1986 act received an average sentence of 10 years and six months. That sentence was longer on average than those given to defendants convicted of weapons offenses (average sentence seven years and seven months) and rape (six years and seven months) and only slightly shorter than the average sentence given to convicted murderers (12 years and nine months). Despite these criticisms, the mandatory minimum sentencing guidelines established in the 1986 act are still in force today.

CONTINUING QUESTIONS

Since its introduction to the United States, crack has been one of the most dangerous and controversial of all drugs. While there is no dispute as to the dangers of using crack, reactions to the drug by lawmakers and law enforcement officials have caused considerable concern among those concerned with the rights of defendants and racial discrimination in sentencing for drug offenses. However, disagreements about the appropriate response to crack use cannot overshadow the fact that crack can lead to serious physical and behavioral problems for the user. The crack epidemic that began in the early 1980s is still claiming victims today.

See also: Dependence and Addiction; Drugs and Criminal Activity; Gangs and Drugs; Illegal Drugs, Common; Law on Drugs, The; Morbidity and Mortality

FURTHER READING

Bayer, Linda N. and Steven L. Jaffe. *Crack & Cocaine (Junior Drug Awareness)*. London, UK: Chelsea House Publications, 2000.

Cooper, Edith Fairman. *The Emergence of Crack Cocaine Abuse*. New York: Novinka Books, 2002.

Karch, Steven B. *A Brief History of Cocaine*. Boca Raton, FL: CRC Press, 1997.

Reinarman, Craig and Harry Gene Levine. *Crack in America: Demon Drugs and Social Justice*. Berkeley: University of California Press, 1997.

■ DEPENDENCE AND ADDICTION

Dependence, the craving for and the compulsive use of a drug despite harmful psychological, physical, or social consequences; and addiction, the inability to stop using a substance despite significant negative physical or psychological effects. No one can predict exactly when a person becomes dependent on a drug because of the many variables involved. Dependence is a very individual situation and it affects people from all walks of life. Its severity varies with the individual, the situation, and the substance. The National Institute on Drug Addiction points out that other issues, such as poor mental health, illness, and occupational or social problems can affect one's ability to overcome a dependency.

Why would a teen choose to take drugs? The truth is that teens may initiate drug use for a variety of reasons. Some of those reasons may include peer pressure, avoiding a difficult family situation, escaping from an abusive relationship, overcoming fears of not meeting expectations, a longing to be accepted in a group, or simple curiosity. Many teens may struggle with some or all of these issues. However, since drug dependence often stems from such difficult emotional or psychological issues, the two need to be dealt with together.

TYPES OF DEPENDENCE

There are several different types and levels of drug dependence. **Physical dependence** occurs when a person comes to depend on a drug to function physically or psychologically. A person who is physically dependent on a drug typically experiences **withdrawal** symptoms when they stop using the substance. These might include nervousness, irritability, trembling, nausea, and even false or distorted sensations known as **hallucinations**. Repeated use of a drug can lead to **tolerance**, a condition in which the user requires ever larger doses of the drug to produce the desired effect.

Q & A

Question: Which drugs have the greatest potential for abuse?

Answer: According to the National Institute on Drug Abuse, almost 70 percent of the people who said they had tried alcohol at least once had used it within a month of the study. Just under 30 percent of those who had experimented with marijuana had smoked it within the previous month.

Not all drugs produce physical dependence. A person also can crave a drug without developing a tolerance for it. **Psychological dependence** is the term for an intense craving for a drug that may or may not be accompanied by physical dependence. When physical and psychological dependence begins to negatively affect a person's life, it is called addiction. Someone who shows three or more of the following behaviors during the same 12-month period is considered addicted:

- Taking larger and larger amounts of the drug
- Taking the drug for a longer period than intended
- Unsuccessful efforts to cut down or control use despite a strong desire to do so
- Spending a great deal of time trying to obtain or use the substance, or recovering from its effects
- Reducing or giving up important activities such as work, school, or recreation because of use
- Continuing to use the drug even though doing so causes physical or psychological problems or makes existing problems worse

The potential for dependence or addiction is related to the physical and psychological properties of the individual drug. Some drugs, including **heroin, LSD, PCP, cocaine,** opium, and **marijuana** can easily lead to psychological dependence. Some of these, particularly cocaine, opium, and heroin, also have a high potential for physical dependence. Other drugs have a lower potential for physical dependence, but all can result in psychological dependence and addiction.

TEENS SPEAK

My Best Friend Got Hooked on Drugs

When Joe got hooked on drugs, I was really ticked off. I knew he smoked cigarettes and had tried some "weed" occasionally but I never thought he would try crack cocaine, let alone get hooked on it.

We both knew about gateway drugs and how using cigarettes or drinking beer can lead to more dangerous drug use, but we never thought it would happen to us. After all, we never did drugs. What really makes me angry is that he never talked with me about it and we were best friends. We shared so much together. Maybe he never talked to me about it because he knew how much I despised drugs. I would tell him that people who use drugs are playing Russian roulette and eventually they will get burned.

Joe would tell me about these kids he knew who would go to raves and do drugs like X, Special K, and even coke. He told me that these guys used these drugs and never had any problems. But I know kids who did drugs at the raves were having trouble at home and in school.

Joe never realized that some of these kids who used drugs at the raves actually ended up in the hospital because they were drinking while taking drugs. I know these club drugs can cause problems but with alcohol they become really dangerous. One guy even attempted suicide. I heard one of the teachers say that this guy was having some problems with depression because his parents were breaking up and that the drugs and alcohol could have prompted the suicide attempt. I hope Joe's okay.

CODEPENDENCE

When a teen is addicted, the drug becomes the single greatest source of pleasure in his or her life. Getting an addicted teen off drugs requires denying him or her this pleasure. This process can be so difficult that professional assistance is required to beat the habit. Drug dependence does not usually happen overnight but rather is the result of a progression of use over time. However, the progression of drug dependence not only involves the users themselves but also their families and friends.

Family and friends can become codependent. **Codependence** is a set of compulsive behaviors learned by persons close to an addict in order to survive in an emotionally painful and stressful environment. People who are codependent often behave in ways that unconsciously support the addict's habit. They may even actively hinder the addict's attempt to beat his or her addiction. Codependent friends or loved ones build their own self-esteem by supporting and caring for the addict. They fear that, without the addiction, he or she may not need them and may even abandon them.

Codependence springs from a person's inability to take care of his or her own emotional needs and a failure to set appropriate emotional boundaries. The codependent person tries to control the feelings and behaviors of others, which can lead to taking responsibility for another person's drug dependence. At the same time, people who are codependent ignore their own needs and wishes. As a result they may experience other psychological problems, including developing addictive behaviors. Because codependence is a mental disorder, treatment is often required to face these problems.

Children exposed to an environment marked by drug dependence and codependence are at risk of modeling the behaviors they witness. They may imitate the behavior of the drug addict and experiment initially with substances like alcohol, cigarettes, or marijuana. These are **gateway drugs**, substances that can lead to the use of increasingly addictive drugs. Some children may copy the behaviors of the codependent family member. Modeling codependence may result in a self-defeating situation, in which children question their personal identity, disregard their feelings, and rely on ineffective coping skills.

Codependence is an example of how drug dependence can affect not only the drug user but also his or her family and friends. It also shows just how difficult it can be to deal with drug dependence. If you think you know someone who may be using drugs, it is much better to approach them before they become dependent. By offering support you can help them avoid making the mistake of becoming involved with drugs.

See also: Drug Abuse, Causes of; Families, Communities, and Drug Abuse; Peer Pressure and Drugs

■ DEPRESSION AND DRUGS

Depression, a mental condition caused by a chemical imbalance in the brain, characterized by feelings of profound sadness, hopelessness, and worthlessness. In 2000, the National Institute of Mental Health (NIMH) estimated that one in every 12 adolescents suffered from depression. When teens suffer setbacks or frustrations in meeting challenges, they may feel depressed. Typically these feelings last only a limited period of time and diminish quickly. However, when feelings of sadness and hopelessness persist and become increasing difficult to overcome, these feelings may indicate the onset of depression. Depression can be treated with **prescription drugs** that are safe and effective. However, some teens turn to illegal drugs or alcohol to deal with their depression. They do not understand the difference between healthy and unhealthy ways of dealing with depression.

SYMPTOMS AND RISK FACTORS

Feeling down is a normal reaction to experiences that result in sadness, disappointment, and rejection. Screwing up on an important exam, needing to put your pet down because of illness, or having your job application rejected are all situations that can leave you feeling blue. However, even when confronted with a terrible tragedy like the untimely death of a loved one, the human spirit usually begins the process of healing and hope, including the feeling that better times are ahead.

When sad feelings persist and begin to affect one's ability to function normally, then a serious condition called depression may be setting in. Depression is characterized by a wide range of feelings that may include dejection, focus on negative thoughts, guilt, low self-esteem, hopelessness, inability to concentrate, loss of appetite, withdrawal from friends, insomnia, and lack of interest in favorite activities. Depression often develops into a cycle in which feelings of worthlessness, helplessness, and loss of control are continually reinforced. A particularly cruel aspect of depression is that it can return unexpectedly when a person is exposed to stressful or difficult situations.

Q & A

Question: How do I know if I am depressed?

Answer: The Web site Psychology Information Online identifies symptoms of depression in teens. If a teen has shown several of these symptoms over several weeks, or if the symptoms cause a significant change in daily life, the teen should talk to someone who can help. The symptoms include:

- Feeling sad or crying often; the sadness doesn't go away
- Feeling guilty for no reason; losing confidence
- Deciding that life seems meaningless or feeling as if nothing good will happen again
- Having a negative attitude much of the time or feeling numb
- No longer doing things one used to like such as music, sports, being with friends, or going out; wanting to be left alone most of the time

- Having trouble making up one's mind; forgetting things and having difficulty concentrating
- Getting irritated often; losing one's temper over little things; overreacting
- Sleeping more or having trouble falling asleep at night; waking up early in the morning and being unable to go back to sleep
- Losing one's appetite or eating a lot more
- Feeling restless and tired
- Thinking about death; feeling as if one is dying; having thoughts about committing suicide

A number of factors can increase one's risk of depression. Some of these factors are related to biology, while others are related to the environment. Some recent research has focused on the hormonal or endocrine system—a system of small glands that regulate bodily functions through hormones released into the bloodstream. Hormones are chemical substances produced in the body. They regulate reaction to stress and sexual development. A 1999 report in the *Journal of Endocrinology* titled "The Role of Corticotropin-Releasing Factor in Depression and Anxiety Disorders" suggests that imbalances in the hormonal system may cause depression. Conditions caused by hormonal imbalances that can lead to depression include Cushing's disease, Addison's disease, and disorders of the thyroid gland.

Chronic (long-term) disease can also be a risk factor for depression. The National Cancer Institute reports that about 25 percent of cancer patients suffer from depression. A 2001 report by the Mayo Clinic found that about the same percentage of diabetes sufferers also experience depression. Other chronic medical conditions that may increase the risk of depression include vitamin deficiency, Parkinson's disease, kidney disease, arthritis, HIV, AIDS, and chronic pain.

Environmental causes for depression can include both negative experiences and ongoing stress. The NIMH reported in 2004 that people who experience more difficulties in childhood are at greater risk of becoming depressed than those who do not suffer as many childhood setbacks. Traumatic experiences such as the death of a loved one, loss of a job, or the end of a relationship can cause a great deal of stress, which may lead to depression. Although research has not proven that stress directly causes depression, those who experience higher levels of stress seem to be at a higher risk for developing depression than those who do not.

Certain psychological disorders can also lead to depression. For example, some people suffer from a condition known as **bipolar disorder,** a mental disorder that causes unusual shifts in mood, energy, and ability to function; people affected with the disorder experience periods of euphoria followed by periods of extreme depression. Depression can also be caused by the lack of sunlight experienced during the winter months especially in the northern sections of the country. This condition—known as seasonal affective disorder, or SAD—can be remedied with special lighting or by packing up and moving to sunnier destinations.

TREATING DEPRESSION

How can you assist a friend who may be depressed? One simple thing you can do is to encourage your friend to seek appropriate medical or psychological help. You may also want to advise him or her to avoid using illegal drugs or alcohol, which can make the symptoms of depression even worse.

Fact Or Fiction?

A positive attitude can pull a teen out of depression.

Fact: Depression is not just a short-term reaction to a temporary disappointment. It is a serious medical condition that can be caused by many factors including stress, chronic disease, and drug or alcohol abuse. Research has shown that optimistic people are healthier than pessimistic ones, and that pessimism is related to depression. However, there is no evidence that pessimism causes depression or that optimism relieves it. Overcoming depression requires counseling and medication.

Some teens feel that illicit drugs and alcohol are helpful in overcoming feelings of sadness and hopelessness. They hope that "getting high" will lift their spirits. There are serious concerns with taking drugs and alcohol to deal with depression. The first is that alcohol and some drugs, such as barbiturates, are **depressants**. Their use can intensify feelings of depression rather than help relieve them. In addition, drinking to cope with depression can often lead to later problems with alcohol and drug abuse.

Another concern is that alcohol and drugs only mask the problem. When their effects wear off, the problem is still there. Sooner or later more alcohol or drugs will be needed to counter feelings of depression.

A variety of legal drugs are available to help people in overcoming their depression. Because researchers believe that depression is caused by a chemical imbalance in the brain, they have developed medications known as **antidepressants** to restore that balance. These antidepressants include Prozac, Luvox, and Zoloft. Another type of medication, Lithium (also produced under the brand names Eskalith and Lithane), is often prescribed for those with a bipolar disorder. Medication in conjunction with therapy can successfully treat most forms of depression.

SUICIDE

Suicide is the act of taking one's own life. It is often the result of long periods of depression. In a 2001 study, the Centers for Disease Control and Prevention reported that suicide was one of the leading causes of deaths among 10- to 24-year-olds.

A study of data collected by the U.S. National Comorbidity Survey during the early 1990s found that people who were dependent on drugs or alcohol were more likely to attempt suicide. The study noted that drug use, even without dependence, was closely associated with suicidal thoughts and impulsive suicide attempts. All drugs seemed equally likely to cause suicidal feelings or attempts.

What teens who attempt suicide often fail to consider is that there is almost always a solution to their problem. Time is a great healer, but suicide robs a person of that valuable time. Feelings of hopelessness may seem impossible to overcome but working through problems can instill a renewed self-confidence. Seeking professional help, staying away from illegal drugs and alcohol, and avoiding negative self-talk are all positive steps in overcoming depression.

See also: Drugs and Drinking; Morbidity and Mortality

■ DRIVING UNDER THE INFLUENCE OF DRUGS

Operating a motor vehicle while impaired by drugs or alcohol. Learning to drive is tough, especially as the roads become increasingly congested with cars, trucks, traffic signals, and pedestrians. It's even more difficult to drive safely with all the distractions of the modern world, including cell phones. The one thing, however, that makes driving not only tough but also extremely dangerous is driving while using alcohol or drugs. Trying to drive under the influence of these substances can even kill you and others.

RATES OF INJURIES AND DEATHS

Teens in the United States are more likely to be killed as the result of a motor-vehicle crash than by any other single activity. Although little is known about what percentage of teens drive under the influence of drugs, the statistics for the percentage of teenagers who drive after drinking alcohol are well established. According to the Centers for Disease Control and Prevention (CDC), in 2001 roughly 13 percent of teens nationwide drove a car or other vehicle after drinking. The rate for males (17 percent) is significantly higher than the rates for females (9.5 percent). Seniors are more likely to drink and drive than juniors, juniors more likely than sophomores, and sophomores more likely than freshman.

Drinking and driving behaviors seem to vary by sex and ethnicity. White males (15 percent) and Hispanic males (13 percent) in the 12th grade were shown to have the highest rates of driving after drinking. By contrast, the rate for African-American males was just under 8 percent. Females were significantly less likely to drink and drive than males, with about 11 percent of white females and 10.5 percent of Hispanic females engaging in such behavior. African-American females (just over 3 percent) were the least likely of all groups to drink and drive. Additionally, the CDC found that about 31 percent of teens nationwide had been a passenger in a car driven by someone who had been drinking alcohol.

Fact Or Fiction?

Seat belts don't prevent injuries.

Fact: In 2000, 80 percent of the teen drivers who were killed in motor vehicle crashes after drinking and driving were not wearing seat belts. Overall, some 14 percent never or rarely wear seat belts when another person is driving. The CDC statistics from 2002 also show that almost twice as many male students as females (18 percent compared to 10 percent) rarely or never wear seat belts.

The National Highway Traffic Safety Administration reported in 2000 that 30 percent of older teen drivers (age 15–20) who died in motor vehicle crashes had been drinking. A 1997 CDC study reported that 14 percent of older teen drivers who died in auto crashes were **legally drunk**, defined as a blood alcohol concentration of 0.10 g/dL (grams of alcohol per deciliter of blood).

A number of factors contribute to teenage alcohol-related fatal motor vehicle crashes, including the time of day, day of the week, and driving experience. The hours between 12 midnight and 3 A.M. are the time of greatest potential risk for an accident. Also, the risk of being killed on a weekend is significantly higher than on a weekday. According to the U.S. Department of Transportation, most alcohol-related fatal motor vehicle crashes occur at night and on the weekends.

The use of **marijuana** and other drugs has also been found to affect the ability of teens to drive safely. In a 1996 study by the National Institute on Drug Abuse (NIDA), researchers found that marijuana impairs functions like balance and coordination, which are essential to safe driving. A compounding problem is driving under the influence of both marijuana and alcohol. NIDA researchers point out that a large number of people who test positive for alcohol also test positive for THC (the active ingredient in marijuana), making it difficult to determine the actual role each drug plays in motor vehicle crashes. A 1994 study conducted by the parliament of the Australian state of Victoria found that drugs other than alcohol were a potential factor in 5 percent of all fatal crashes. The study showed that 11 percent of driver fatalities involved the use of marijuana, about 4 percent involved **stimulants** (drugs that stimulate the central nervous system) and another 3 percent involved **opiates** (drugs that depress the central nervous system).

Q & A

Question: How much alcohol intake impairs one's ability to drive?

Answer: The law defines drunk as having a blood alcohol concentration (BAC) of 0.10 grams of alcohol per deciliter of blood (g/dL). However, according to the counseling services department of the University of Wisconsin at Eau Claire, considerably smaller doses of alcohol can impair driving skills:

- At 0.02 g/dL, light to moderate drinkers begin to feel the intoxicating effects of alcohol

- At 0.04 g/dL, most people start to feel relaxed
- At 0.06 g/dL, most people are less able to make a rational decision about their ability to drive
- At 0.08 g/dL, muscle coordination and driving skills are clearly impaired
- At 0.10 g/dL, your reaction time and ability to control a car deteriorate rapidly (this is legally drunk in all states)

A 160-pound male who consumes five drinks over a three-hour period will have a BAC of about .76. A 140-pound female who consumes four drinks in the same time will have a BAC of .80.

LEGAL ISSUES

Accidents are the most obvious danger associated with driving while on drugs, but driving after using drugs or alcohol can result in legal problems as well. A teen who is convicted of DUI—driving under the influence of drugs or alcohol—will usually lose his or her license for six months to a year. Younger teen drivers may have the conviction erased from their record after completing various judicial requirements including attending traffic school, learning about alcohol abuse, and parole. However, if a DUI conviction cannot be removed from one's record, it becomes a permanent mark that could impact future employment opportunities. Some employers will not hire people who have a DUI on their record. Other potential employers may view the infraction as an indication of poor decision-making skills and hire someone with a clean record.

Can a teen be cited for DUI if he or she was not driving drunk? Even if teens do not drive under the influence they can still be arrested for underage drinking and driving. The penalties may vary according to a variety of factors, including local and state ordinances, prior convictions, willingness to cooperate, and other circumstances surrounding the event. Often underage drinking and driving will result in the temporary loss of driving privileges.

According to a 2003 CDC study, alcohol-related traffic fatalities among older teens declined from 5,504 in 1992 to 2,442 in 2002. However the CDC states that about 1.4 million arrests for DUI are still made yearly. In the future, increased efforts to prevent teen alcohol related motor-vehicle crashes might include:

- Suspending the driver's licenses of those driving while intoxicated
- Lowering the permissible levels of blood alcohol for adults to 0.08 g/dL and zero tolerance for those under 21
- Establishing sobriety checkpoints where police stop drivers to check for those who may be driving while under the influence
- Continued public education and media campaigns

The most important preventative measure, however, is one's own judgment. The best first step is to avoid alcohol and illegal drugs altogether. Those who do drink or use drugs should never drive while under the influence. No one should ride with a driver that he or she knows or suspects is under the influence of drugs. If you know someone who has been drinking or using drugs, try to prevent them from driving; perhaps you can even offer to drive them home. Keep in mind that driving, drugs, and alcohol never mix well.

See also: Drugs and Drinking; Law on Drugs, The; Morbidity and Mortality

■ DRUG ABUSE, CAUSES OF

The nonmedical use of a substance in order to affect one's mental processes, satisfy a **dependence** (an intense physical or psychological need for a substance), or attempt suicide. Nonmedical means that use of the drug was not prescribed by a medical professional (such as a doctor, a dentist, a nurse practitioner, or a pharmacist). If a person takes a **prescription drug** that was prescribed for someone else, he or she is also engaging in nonmedical use of a substance. If a person doubles the prescribed dosage of a painkiller, he or she is also engaging in nonmedical use of a drug. So are those who take an over-the-counter cough suppressant without following the instructions on the label.

Not all nonmedical use of drugs is drug abuse. In order for a nonmedical use to be classified as drug abuse, the user must intend to affect the way his or her brain functions, satisfy a previously established drug dependence, or attempt suicide.

What causes people to abuse drugs? What leads one teenager to experiment with drugs and another to refuse to have anything to do with drugs? What leads one experimenter to abuse drugs for years and another to quickly outgrow his or her interest in experimentation? Many scientists do not agree on the answers to those questions. Some believe the answer lies in a person's genetics, the study of how particular qualities or traits are passed from parents to their offspring. Other scientists believe the answer lies in one's environment, or surroundings. Those scientists examine aspects of family life, culture, and society that appear to increase the likelihood that a person will abuse drugs.

Q & A

Question: Are adolescent males more likely to use drugs than adolescent females?

Answer: Gender makes a big difference. Among males over age 12, 12.8 percent are likely to be classified as dependent on or abusing drugs. Among females over age 12, the percentage drops to 6.1 percent. Among teens between the ages of 12 and 17, however, the difference is not nearly as significant—9.3 percent of the male population and 8.6 percent of the female population abuse drugs.

Most likely, a combination of factors causes drug abuse. Four factors that have especially interested social scientists are **social skills**, psychological health, family and peers, and society.

SOCIAL SKILLS
Social scientists define social skills as the behaviors that determine whether one is popular, accepted by his or her peers, and liked by family members and authority figures (such as teachers). Individuals acquire—and fine-tune—social skills throughout their lives, but childhood and adolescence are crucial to their acquisition. The degree to which teens master social skills may affect any number of behaviors. Research indicates, for example, that teenagers who have not succeeded in establishing good relations with their peers are more likely than other teenagers to do poorly in school, cut classes, engage in delinquent behavior, hang around with peers who get into trouble, drop out of school—and abuse drugs. Children with attention deficit disorder—an inability to concentrate on a task for sustained periods of

time—and those who exhibit aggressive-impulsive behavior, such as striking out suddenly and violently with little provocation, are also at greater risk of abusing drugs.

It is important to understand, however, that being at risk of abusing drugs does not mean one will actually become a drug abuser. Being at risk means that researchers have found statistical evidence linking one thing (in this case, deficient social skills) with another thing (in this case, drug abuse) in a significant number of cases. Many other factors—including teacher or parental involvement in one's life, or one's ability and determination to assess a situation and weigh its consequences—can reduce the likelihood of abuse.

On the other hand, deficient social skills can snowball. Teenagers with deficient social skills may find themselves isolated or accepted only by other teenagers in the same situation. Gangs hold particular attraction to such teens, and in gangs drug use may be the expectation. Using drugs may seem to alleviate the pain of social rejection, so much so that it turns into abuse.

Researchers seeking to minimize the incidence of drug abuse among teenagers have created programs that teach social skills. In particular, teenagers learn to evaluate the medical and social consequences of drug use. They also learn the dynamics of peer acceptance, and how to assert themselves in the face of peer pressure. (One's peers are people of the same age and social group.)

PSYCHOLOGICAL HEALTH

Not surprisingly, researchers have found a statistical relationship between serious emotional and behavioral problems and drug abuse. As noted previously, teenagers with attention deficits are more likely than other teenagers to abuse drugs.

In 1999, the Substance Abuse and Mental Health Services Administration (SAMHSA), an agency of the Department of Health and Human Services, released a study titled "The Relationship Between Mental Health and Substance Abuse Among Adolescents." The authors reported that teenagers who have chronic (long-term) difficulty concentrating on schoolwork, on chores at home, work, and even sports activities may be experiencing depression or the early signs of a **mental illness**. For such teenagers, drug use is a seemingly attractive answer to problems that feel insurmountable. The emotional distress that naturally results from school failure, family discord, and neighborhood violence may also lead a teenager to seek comfort in drugs.

On the other hand, drug use and drug abuse can cause or exacerbate (increase or heighten) psychological difficulties. Sometimes a teenager will use drugs to counteract the symptoms of depression even though drugs can trigger depression or deepen it. Similarly, one teen may abuse drugs in response to school failure, while another teenager may experience school failure after drug abuse overtakes his or her life.

The SAMHSA study found that teenagers whose psychological problems resulted in behaviors like stealing, showing physical aggression, or running away from home were seven times more likely to abuse drugs or alcohol than were teenagers who had minimal or no emotional problems. The psychologically troubled teenagers were nearly nine times as likely as their minimally troubled or untroubled peers to need treatment for drug abuse.

Early intervention (action by others to help resolve a problem) is the key. The SAMHSA study reports that two-thirds of young people in the United States with diagnosable mental disorders do not get help. If family members, teachers, health-care professionals, and friends recognize signs of psychological distress or depression in a teenager, they should get help for him or her. In so doing, they may be able to save that person from emotional turmoil and the consequences of drug abuse.

FAMILY AND PEERS

Researchers have wondered about the degree to which the influence of parents and peers determines a teenager's use and abuse of drugs. They have also asked whether parents or peers are the more influential. The authors of "Parental Influences on Adolescent Marijuana Use and the Baby Boom Generation," a SAMHSA study released in 2001, report that parental influence may be far stronger than was previously thought.

The SAMHSA study noted that parents' *attitudes* toward drug use (in this case, **marijuana** use) were far more influential than the parents' own *experiences* with drugs.

Fact Or Fiction?

Children whose mothers smoke cigarettes and use alcohol are more likely to abuse drugs than children whose fathers do so.

Fact: The 2001 SAMHSA report "Parental Influences of Adolescent Marijuana Use and the Baby Boom Generation" declares that cigarette smoking and alcohol use by fathers had no impact on their children's substance use. In contrast, mothers' cigarette smoking and alcohol use had a significant influence. Children whose mothers smoked cigarettes and used alcohol were likely to be lifetime users of marijuana.

From an early age, long before they have much exposure to their peers, children pick up on their parents' attitudes toward drugs. They not only observe how their parents use a variety of substances—prescribed drugs, over-the-counter medications, nicotine (in cigarettes), alcohol—but also listen to the way their parents talk about these substances. They also evaluate the extent to which their parents' actions match their words. Not surprisingly, teens whose parents abuse drugs or alcohol are significantly more likely to abuse drugs or alcohol themselves.

What role, then, do peers play in drug abuse by teenagers? According to those social scientists that believe drug use is a learned behavior, peers play a significant role. Those researchers contend that a person comes to abuse drugs by copying, or modeling, the behaviors of those around him or her, including drug abuse. When someone takes a drug for the first time and receives positive reinforcement from friends for doing so or acceptance by a perceived in-group, he or she is encouraged to continue the behavior.

TEENS SPEAK

At the First Dance of the Year

I'm Billy. My friend Bobby and I were disappointed when summer ended, but we were looking forward to the first school dance of the year. School dances are lame, but they're something to do, and the first one of the school year is a way of catching up with everybody after the summer. So Bobby and I went to the dance.

When we saw some of our buddies heading outside, Bobby and I joined them. Everybody was talking about a rave downtown. Justin, a senior, had his mother's car. He piled a bunch of kids into the car and headed downtown.

Everyone in the car yelled for the rest of us to come too. Bobby and I looked at each other, and we both nodded at the same time. I have my own car, an SUV. So I got it and drove back to pick up the rest of the gang.

I'd never been to a rave before. It was way cool. Bobby and I were digging the music. Then, without warning, one of our buddies gave Bobby and me each a white tablet. I looked closely. The letters *XTC* were printed on mine.

Our buddy said, "Take this, and you'll party all night."

Bobby wasn't sure. He was looking to me for guidance. He said, "Should we?"

Our buddy was reassuring. He said, "It won't hurt you. All that happens is that you won't need to eat or drink or sleep for a while."

I started feeling uncomfortable. It bothered me to take something I really didn't know anything about. Bobby looked at me again, but now he was excited. He said, "Let's try it."

So I was squirming. I didn't want to be a wimp, but I also didn't want to get screwed up on some crazy drug. Then I thought of a way out. "Thanks, but I'm driving," I said to our buddy. I didn't want Bobby taking it either, so I said to him, "I have to get the car back, or I'll be grounded for the rest of the millennium." An excellent move. I grabbed Bobby and we got out of there.

In a way, I would've liked to have stayed. The rave was cool. But I think it's stupid to take a drug you know nothing about just because some guy who's probably already high recommends it. Besides, Bobby and I hardly knew the guy. No. I have too much respect for myself—and my life—for that.

Related to both parental influence and peer influence is the family's socioeconomic status—how much education parents have had and how much income the family has. According to SAMHSA's report on the results of the 2002 National Survey on Drug Use and Health, less-educated adults were more likely to abuse drugs than college graduates. As for employment—an important indicator of family income—10.6 percent of adults working full-time suffered from drug dependence; 10.5 percent of those working part-time were drug dependent; and 19.7 percent of those who were unemployed were drug dependent.

Where one lives matters, too. According to the 2002 survey, among persons over age 12 the rate of substance dependence or abuse was 9.3 percent for those in large metropolitan areas, 10.1 percent for those in small metropolitan areas, 8.3 percent for those in nonmetropolitan areas (smaller towns), and just 6.5 percent for those in rural areas. In the country overall, the rate of substance dependence or abuse also varies: it is 10.2 percent in the Midwest, 9.6 percent in the West, 9 percent in the South, and 8.7 percent in the Northeast.

SOCIETY

A society is an enduring group of human beings distinguished from other groups by mutual interests, shared institutions (such as government education, media), and a common culture or way of life. The society in which one lives is an environmental factor that may influence drug abuse.

Is society a *cause* of drug abuse? Does it lead its members to use and abuse drugs? Society in itself—especially a society as diverse as that of the United States—is too large to be studied as a whole, or to be blamed for its members' drug abuse. Yet clearly drug abuse is a problem in American society (and in other societies throughout the world).

Drugs are prevalent in American society, and so drug abuse presents a viable option to many Americans, especially teenagers. If one can obtain drugs easily, he or she can use them and abuse them. Drugs—legal and illegal drugs, prescribed and over-the-counter drugs—are all prevalent in American popular culture.

See also: Depression and Drugs; Families, Communities, and Drug Abuse; Over-the-Counter Drugs; Risk Factors and Risk Taking; School Performance and Drug Abuse

FURTHER READING

Muisener, Philip. *Understanding and Treating Adolescent Substance Abuse.* Thousand Oaks, CA: Sage Publications, Inc., 1994.

Walters, Glenn D. *Escaping the Journey to Nowhere: The Psychology of Alcohol and Other Drug Abuse.* Bristol, PA: Taylor & Francis, 1994.

■ DRUG COUNSELING
See: Depression and Drugs; Rehabilitation and Treatment

■ DRUG LAWS
See: Law on Drugs, The

■ DRUG TESTS
See: Workplace Drug Abuse

■ DRUG VICTIMS
See: Homicide; Morbidity and Mortality

■ DRUG USE, HISTORY OF
The medical and recreational use and abuse of drugs is not a new phenomenon. Naturally occurring drugs such as **opium** and **marijuana** have been used almost since the beginning of recorded history. With the advance of science and medical technology, humans have also invented synthetic drugs such as **amphetamines** and **ecstasy**. Additionally, some of today's best-known drugs, including **cocaine** and **heroin**, were created by using modern scientific processes to chemically alter natural substances that have been known for centuries.

MARIJUANA
According to the National Institute on Drug Abuse, marijuana is the most widely used illicit drug in the United States. Marijuana was not always illegal. It has been widely used for recreational, medical, and commercial purposes. Interestingly, in some places where marijuana was used commercially and medically, it never gained popularity as an intoxicating drug. In other places, intoxication was its principal use.

In 1972, the National Commission on Marihuana and Drug Abuse presented a report to Congress titled "Marihuana, A Signal of Misunderstanding," which traced a detailed history of marijuana from ancient times to the early 1970s. According to the report, some of the earliest references to marijuana appear in a Chinese medical text dated 2737 B.C. The Chinese emperor Shen-Nung recommended it as a treatment for the nutritional disease beriberi, constipation, "female weakness," gout, malaria, rheumatism, and "absentmindedness." However, the Chinese appear not to have used marijuana as an intoxicant.

From China, marijuana seems to have spread south and west to India, where it became a major part of Hindu culture by 1000 B.C. In India, marijuana was called the "Giver of Life." Hindus who were in the highest social caste, or class, were not permitted to use alcohol but could freely use marijuana. Thus, high-caste Hindus included the drug (which they called *bhang*) in religious ceremonies as well as at marriage celebrations and family festivals. The working classes in India came to regard marijuana in much the same way people in Europe and the United States viewed beer. They smoked bhang and drank it in a liquid form at the end of the day to relieve stress and fatigue. According to one source cited in the report, Indians used marijuana "to obtain a sense of well-being, to stimulate appetite, and to enable them to bear more cheerfully the strain and monotony of daily routines"

India was not the only part of central Asia where marijuana gained popularity at this time. Clay tablet inscriptions found in present-day Iran show that the drug was used there around 700–600 B.C. Records from the Mesopotamian empire of Assyria indicate its use at the time of King Ashurbanipal's reign (669–626 B.C.).

From central Asia and the Middle East, the drug spread to Greece. In his epic story the *Odyssey*, the great Greek author Homer describes a drug called *nepenthe,* which many scholars believe was a liquid brew in which the most active ingredient was marijuana. The ancient Romans also employed marijuana as an intoxicant, according to the Roman author and physician Galen. In the second century A.D. Galen recorded that Romans would often serve marijuana to guests at banquets "to promote hilarity and happiness." Marijuana was also popular in the early Muslim world. Like upper-caste Hindus, devout Muslims were not allowed to drink alcohol. Long before 1000 A.D. the drug not only appeared in the Muslim world but also became a part of Muslim culture.

Records indicate that marijuana was used medically in Africa long before it became popular as an intoxicant. Texts from Egypt dating to the 1900s B.C. show that it was used to treat sore eyes. Marijuana was used in other parts of Africa as an antiseptic and to restore appetite and relieve hemorrhoidal pain. Other medical uses for marijuana included the treatment of tetanus, rabies, convulsion in infants, nervous disorders, cholera, rheumatism, hay fever, asthma, skin diseases, and difficult labor during childbirth.

Aside from its use in ancient Greece and Rome, most Europeans had never heard of marijuana until the 1800s. Muslims apparently brought the drug to Spain in the 900s A.D., but its use did not spread beyond the Muslim community. Some scholars believe that the Italian explorer Marco Polo may have known about marijuana before his famous trip to China in the 1200s. They are convinced that he encountered a powerful and concentrated form of marijuana called hashish when he journeyed through the Middle East during his travels.

Marijuana seems to have first gained some popularity in Europe as a result of French emperor Napoleon Bonaparte's invasion of Egypt in the early 1800s. Two scientific reports prepared later in the century further increased European interest in marijuana. In 1839, the British physician W. B. O'Shaughnessy recommended the medical use of marijuana for a variety of illnesses and as a mild intoxicant. A later report by Russell Reynolds, the private physician to England's Queen Victoria, made many of the same recommendations. Members of Europe's medical profession during the mid-1800s spoke highly of the drug, which was easily obtained without a prescription.

Many popular writers of the day, including Charles Baudelaire, Arthur Rimbaud, and Pierre Gautier, wrote enthusiastically about the effects of hashish. Gautier and Baudelaire were even members of the Club des Hachischins, in which writers and intellectuals gathered and experimented with hashish. Although intrigued by the writers' descriptions of their experiences with the drug, the public at large looked upon marijuana with a mix of fear and repugnance. As a result, hashish remained a drug whose use was largely confined to a few European artists and intellectuals.

Historians disagree as to when marijuana first arrived in the United States. Some suggest that the Spanish brought the plant with them during their exploration of the Americas in the 1500s. Others claim that the drug was brought over on slave ships. Yet hemp plant from which the drug is derived has been grown in what is now the United States for centuries, apparently without widespread knowledge of its intoxicating effects. Early Americans used hemp for clothing, rope, and twine, and the first pioneers used hemp cloth to cover their wagons.

During the 1800s, marijuana was often used as a medicine in the United States. Although available without a prescription, it was also widely prescribed by physicians for a variety of ailments. In 1857, the Boston physician John Bell reported using marijuana to control mental and emotional disorders in the mentally ill. Three years later, the Ohio State Medical Society's Committee on Cannabis Indica claimed that its members had used marijuana to successfully treat pain, hemorrhage, hysteria, mania, whooping cough, infantile convulsions, asthma, gonorrhea, nervous rheumatism, chronic bronchitis, muscular spasms, tetanus, and epilepsy. It was also used to stimulate appetite.

The first recorded use of marijuana as an intoxicant in the United States dates to the early 1900s. American soldiers stationed in Puerto Rico and the Panama Canal Zone were using it by 1916. American soldiers fighting the Mexican bandit Pancho Villa also began to smoke marijuana around this time. Marijuana use in the United States grew during the 1910s and 1920s as large numbers of Mexican laborers came north for work and brought the drug with them.

During the 1920s and 1930s, marijuana grew in popularity in the United States, especially among musicians and other entertainers. It was at this time that the federal government began to express concern about the spread of the drug. The first federal antimarijuana laws were passed in the 1930s, in what is considered the beginning of the nation's "war on drugs." One campaign by the Federal Bureau of Narcotics portrayed marijuana as a powerful, addicting substance that would lead users into narcotics addiction. This idea of marijuana as a "gateway" drug is still supported by some authorities. These efforts, however, failed to curb a growing interest in the drug. During the 1950s, it became popular among the so-called beat generation of poets, writers, and musicians. In the 1960s, its use spread to college campuses where it became a symbol of rebellion against authority.

In 1970, the federal government classified marijuana as a Schedule I drug—a drug that has the highest potential for abuse and no accepted medical use. In effect, the government proclaimed marijuana to be as dangerous as heroin or LSD. By the 1980s, the government had adopted a "zero-tolerance" program that resulted in the passage of mandatory prison sentences for possession of marijuana. This period saw a decline in the use of marijuana, a trend which began to reverse itself in the early 1990s. However, by 2000, use of the drug had once again declined below previous levels. According to the 2003 "Monitoring the Future" study, about 46 percent of 12th graders report having tried marijuana, while about 35 percent had used it in the previous year.

COCAINE

According to Arthur Gibson, a University of California–Los Angeles expert on the history of commercial uses of plants, evidence of coca use dates back to 3000 B.C. At that time, the Valdiva people of coastal Ecuador produced figurines and ceramic pots showing individuals chewing coca leaves. Other ceramics showing the use of the stimulant have been found in Peru dating from 1900 to 1750 B.C. In the Nazca region of Peru, 2,000-year-old mummies were found with bags of coca leaves (chuspas) around their necks.

However, the Incan civilization of Peru, which arose around 1300 A.D., provides the earliest useful information about early coca use. For the Incas, coca was a symbol of royalty. Only male royalty, priests, and shamans were allowed to use the drug. Reports also suggest that coca was used to treat the sick and soothe pain from ailments such as toothache and malaria. Court orators used the drug so they could recount Incan history at a single sitting. It was also used during initiation rites for young men. Thus, coca use in Incan society was typically for medical or ceremonial purposes rather than as an intoxicant.

By the time of the Spanish invasion of Peru in 1533 A.D., the power of the ruling class had weakened greatly and coca was no longer a symbol of political or social status. The conquest of the Incas brought Spanish culture and the Roman Catholic Church to South America. Priests who wanted to convert the Indians to Catholicism opposed coca because they associated it with Incan culture and religion. In 1551, the bishop of Cuzco banned its use and called it "an evil agent of the Devil." Anyone using or possessing coca could be burned at the stake. As coca plantations were cut down, the coca leaf business went underground. For many South American Indians, using coca became a way of defying Spanish authority.

In time, the Spanish found that coca was indispensable to their mining operations in the Americas. Under great pressure to increase production of gold and silver, Spain's King Phillip II decreed in 1569 that coca was not evil. Spanish overseers now supplied the Indians with coca leaves to increase their energy and productivity. Even priests who once called the drug evil now said that it was aiding "God's work." At this time, a merchant named Nicolas Monardes tried to import coca leaves to Spain, but they decayed during the long voyage. It was not until the late 1800s that coca enjoyed a revival of interest in Europe. In 1814, some wealthy Londoners wanted to use coca to replace food for the poor so they could increase the productivity of child labor. However, coca leaves were still unavailable in Europe at this time.

In 1860, an Italian physician named Paolo Mantegazza was the first to isolate the active ingredient in coca leaves and produce the drug now called cocaine. About the same time, the chemist Angelo Mariani extracted cocaine from coca leaves and put it into cough drops and wine. His creation, called Mariani's Coca Wine or Dr. Mariani's French Tonic, became extremely popular in Europe and then found fans in the United States. A host of famous and influential people endorsed its use. Pope Leo XIII even gave Mariani a gold medal for inventing a potion that relieved fatigue, lifted the spirits, and gave people a sense of well-being. Cocaine began to appear in popular literature at this time. The famous fictional detective Sherlock Holmes injected cocaine to relieve boredom when he was not working on a case, and Robert Louis Stevenson supposedly wrote the novel *Dr. Jekyll and Mr. Hyde* while under the influence of cocaine.

One of the most enthusiastic supporters of cocaine use was the psychiatrist Sigmund Freud. While searching for a cure for nervous exhaustion and morphine addiction, Freud found that cocaine relieved his own depression, and he wrote a series of papers about the drug, praising it as a "magical drug" superior to morphine. In 1884, Freud recommended the use of cocaine to a Vienna ophthalmologist named Karl Koller as a local anesthetic for eye operations. Koller discovered that cocaine was also useful as an anesthetic for surgery of the ear, nose, and throat.

During the late 1800s and early 1900s, cocaine appeared in many tonics, elixirs, and popular medicines. In 1886, John S. Pemberton invented Coca-Cola by combining caramel, phosphoric acid, an extract of the kola nut that contained caffeine, and cocaine. He added sugar to the formula to disguise the bitterness of the cocaine. Cocaine-based medications were extremely popular in the United States throughout the early 1900s. However, as with marijuana, federal government officials became concerned about the use of the drug. Congress passed laws banning the sale and distribution of cocaine during the 1930s, and like marijuana use, cocaine use went underground.

The use of cocaine as an illegal intoxicant increased during the 1950s and 1960s, but its relatively high price made it less popular than other illicit drugs. By the 1970s, it had become the drug of choice among many wealthy and middle-class drug users. Cocaine retained an image as a more "refined" drug until the 1980s, when a powerful version called crack appeared in the United States. Crack was not only more potent but also considerably cheaper than powder cocaine. An epidemic of crack use in the 1980s, accompanied by gang violence associated with crack dealing, led to stiff penalties for possession and sale of crack. In recent years cocaine and crack use has been on the decline, especially among teens. According to the 2002 "Monitoring the Future" study, about 9 percent of 12th graders had tried cocaine at least once, down from a peak of 17.3 percent in 1985. About 3.8 percent of 12th graders in 2002 reported using crack at some time in their lives, and 2.2 percent had smoked crack in the previous year.

OPIUM AND HEROIN

Opium is one of the oldest drugs known to humans. According to the book *Opium: A History*, by Martin Bloom, opium poppies were grown by the Sumerians of lower Mesopotamia as early as 3400 B.C. They referred to it as the "joy plant." The Sumerians passed the plant along to the Assyrians, who transferred their knowledge of it to the Babylonians, who in turn introduced opium to Egypt. The opium trade flourished during the 1300s and 1200s B.C. Merchants from Phoenicia and Minoa shipped opium to Egypt, Carthage, and Europe.

In the 400s B.C., the Greek physician Hippocrates, known as "the father of medicine," acknowledged that opium was useful as a narcotic as well as for treating internal diseases, diseases of women, and epidemics. Some 100 years later, Alexander the Great brought opium for his armies on their conquest of Persia and India, introducing the drug to parts of the Middle East. By 400 A.D., Arab traders brought the drug to China.

Despite its early introduction to Europe, opium use virtually disappeared in Europe until the 1500s A.D. At that time, Portuguese traders sailing the East China Sea discovered the intoxicating effects of smoking the drug. Although the Portuguese first encountered opium in China, the Chinese themselves considered the practice of smoking the drug barbaric. By 1527, the drug had once again come to the attention of Europeans through medical literature. The Renaissance physician Paracelsus reported on the existence of black pills called laudanum, which were made of opium, citrus juice, and gold extract. Known as "Stones of Immortality," the pills were prescribed as painkillers.

Opium use became widespread in Europe during the 1600s and 1700s. England's Queen Elizabeth I ordered English merchants to bring high-quality opium from India to England, and in 1680 English chemist Thomas Sydenham introduced Sydenham's Laudanum, a compound of opium, sherry wine, and herbs. These and other potions containing opium became popular remedies for numerous ailments.

In 1803, a German chemist named Friedrich Sertuerner discovered the active ingredient of opium. By dissolving opium in acid then neutralizing it with ammonia, he produced morphine, the first synthetic opium-based drug. Many physicians who were wary of using opium because it was so powerful believed that opium had finally been "tamed." Morphine was called "God's own medicine" for its safety, reliability, and long-lasting effects. In 1843, Dr. Alexander Wood of Scotland became the first to inject morphine with a syringe. He found that the effects were almost instantaneous and several times more potent than opium or morphine taken orally. In 1895, German chemist Heinrich Dreser produced a morphine-based drug that did not have many of the common side effects of morphine. The drug, called heroin, was first marketed commercially three years later.

By 1900, opium and morphine use had spread throughout Europe, Asia, and the United States. Their use generated concern, because many users became addicted to the drugs. In the early 1900s, the Saint James Society in the United States began to supply free samples of heroin through the mail to morphine addicts who were trying to give up their habits. However, within a few years, the rate of heroin addiction in the United States had grown alarmingly. In 1905, the U.S. Congress banned the use of opium, and by 1925 all opium-based narcotics were declared illegal in the United States.

The ban, however, did not stop the use of heroin or other opium-based drugs—it merely drove them underground. A thriving black market for the drugs developed, and heroin remained readily available through street dealers in large cities such as New York. In the mid-to-late 1900s, cultivation of opium poppies became a major source of revenue for many rebel groups in Thailand, Burma, Vietnam, and other Asian nations. Profits from opium and heroin cultivation also financed terrorist groups operating out of Afghanistan.

The recreational use of heroin in the United States peaked during the 1960s and 1970s before beginning a gradual decline in the 1980s. Heroin use rose again during the 1990s, and since that time, use by teens has gradually increased. According to the Substance Abuse and

Mental Health Services Administration's National Household Survey on Drug Abuse, the percentage of teens age 12–17 who used heroin rose from 0.1 percent to 0.4 percent between 1995 and 2002. Heroin use by adults age 18–25 rose from 0.8 to 1.6 percent. In 2003, 404,000 Americans age 12 and older reported using heroin during the past year, and 3.7 million reported using it at least once in their lives.

Fact Or Fiction?

Great Britain and China fought wars over opium smuggling.

Fact: Between 1839 and 1856, Great Britain and China engaged in two "opium wars" over the British importation of opium into China. In the late 1700s, the British East India Company discovered a huge market for opium in China, where the drug was illegal except for medicinal purposes. The company made huge profits by smuggling it into China. Angered by the British trade, the Chinese emperor banned all sale and importation of opium in 1799. In 1839, Chinese authorities ordered foreigners to turn over their stores of opium to the government. Unwilling to give up the profitable trade, the British declared war on China. After two years of fighting, the victorious British claimed the Chinese island of Hong Kong as a colony and resumed the opium trade.

The Chinese refused to accept this state of affairs, and hostilities erupted into a second opium war in 1856. This time, the French, who now had colonies in the opium-producing areas of Southeast Asia, joined the British. Once again, the Chinese were defeated, and they were forced to lift the ban on importation of opium into China.

SYNTHETIC DRUGS

Most of today's other widely abused drugs are synthetically produced substances that have had a much briefer history of use. For example, the drug LSD was first created in Switzerland in the 1950s and soon gained a reputation for producing powerful **hallucinations** and other out-of-body experiences. It became popular among college students during the 1960s, largely as a result of the writings and speeches of author Timothy Leary, who encouraged American youths to experiment with the drug under the slogan "turn on, tune in, and drop out."

Amphetamine, another widely used synthetic drug, was first synthesized in Germany in 1887. However, it was not used until the late

1920s, when it was investigated as a cure for a variety of illnesses, including epilepsy, **schizophrenia**, alcoholism, opiate addiction, migraine, head injuries, and radiation sickness. In 1932, amphetamine was marketed as an **over-the-counter** inhaler to treat nasal congestion. Five years later it was found to have a positive effect on some children with attention deficit hyperactivity disorder (ADHD). In 1919, scientists in Japan discovered methamphetamine, which was more potent and easier to make than amphetamine.

During World War II, the U.S. Army used amphetamines to keep soldiers alert and reduce fatigue. After the war, supplies of methamphetamine once used for military purposes were made available to the Japanese. The result was an epidemic of **intravenous** methamphetamine abuse. At the same time, tablets of legally manufactured amphetamine and methamphetamine became readily available in the United States and were used recreationally by college students, truck drivers, and athletes. Abuse of the drugs spread widely and continues to be a major problem today.

Some of the newest synthetic drugs are the so-called club drugs, or designer drugs. Many of these drugs were originally created in the 1970s as treatments for medical conditions. For example, the drug GHB was originally sold as an over-the-counter substance used for weight reduction and to build muscle mass. Users soon became aware of its **sedative** effects and its ability to produce euphoria, leading to widespread abuse. The federal government banned sale of GHB in 1992. The club drug ketamine was first developed as an anesthetic for veterinary medicine, which is still its main medical use. However, ketamine also became a drug of abuse because of its ability to produce euphoria.

The history of drug use and abuse shows that humans have long been fascinated with the medical and recreational uses of drugs. While many drugs have been used primarily as intoxicants, few have gained popularity on that basis alone. Drugs such as heroin, cocaine, and amphetamines were first prized for their curative abilities before they were abused for their intoxicating effects. As shown by the rise in popularity of new substances such as club drugs, humans' fascination with drugs continues today.

See also: Club and Designer Drugs; Crack Cocaine; Drugs and Criminal Activity; Gangs and Drugs; Illegal Drugs, Common; Injection Drugs

FURTHER READING

Booth, Martin. *Opium: A History.* London, UK: Simon and Schuster, Ltd., 1996.

Gahlinger, Paul M. *Illegal Drugs: A Complete Guide to Their History, Chemistry, Use, and Abuse.* Ogden, UT: Sagebrush Press, 2001.

Knowles, Cynthia R. *Up All Night: A Closer Look at Club Drugs and Rave Culture.* Thousand Oaks, CA: Red House Press, 2001.

Tracy, Sarah and Caroline Jean Acker. *Altering American Consciousness: The History of Alcohol and Drug Use in the United States, 1800-2000.* Amherst: University of Massachusetts Press, 2004.

■ DRUGS AND CRIMINAL ACTIVITY

Illegal acts such as theft, assault, homicide, or drug use. When people think of drugs and criminal activity, they often picture gang-related crime associated with dealing drugs. However, while youth gangs are a significant threat to public safety, gang violence represents only a small portion of the criminal activity tied to drug use. According to a fact sheet on drug-related crime published by the Office of National Drug Control Policy (March 2000), drugs are also related to crime through the effects they have on the user's behavior and by generating violence and other illegal activity in conjunction with drug sales. Therefore, domestic violence and school violence are often linked to drug and alcohol use. Often the victims are bystanders who happened to be in the wrong place at the wrong time. However, those who abuse drugs may also frequently fall victim to violence from drug and alcohol abuse. Since the 1980s, drug-related crime has become a major problem for law enforcement officials.

DRUG ABUSERS AS PERPETRATORS OF CRIME

The physical and psychological effects of drugs and alcohol contribute in a variety of ways to the likelihood of criminal activity. Some drugs, such as alcohol, **cocaine** (a highly addictive stimulant), and **amphetamines** (a group of drugs that stimulate the central nervous system) have been shown to increase aggressive tendencies. These and a wide range of other drugs—including **marijuana** (a drug made from hemp that is smoked for its euphoric effect), **heroin** (a powerful painkiller that is highly addictive), and various **prescription drugs**—

can also impair the user's judgment and reduce inhibitions. Under the influence of drugs or alcohol, a person may be much more likely to engage in risk-taking behaviors (such as criminal activity)—behaviors that he or she would probably avoid when sober. In addition, someone who is dependent on a drug or addicted to it may steal to support his or her drug habit.

Type and Incidence of drug-related crimes

The U.S. criminal justice system classifies crimes into two broad categories: property crimes and violent crimes against individuals. Property crimes include larceny, shoplifting, and burglary; crimes against individuals include homicide, domestic violence, and sexual assault. A 1995 report from the National Institute on Drug Abuse (NIDA) defined the extent to which drugs and alcohol are involved in both types of crime. The report "NIDA Refocuses Its Research on Drug-Related Violence" points out that 25–30 percent of violent crimes and 3–4 percent of property crimes are caused by alcohol abuse (a drinking pattern that leads to negative behavior and possibly addiction). Meanwhile, 25–30 percent of property crimes and 4–5 percent of violent crimes can be attributed to illegal drug use.

By definition, using illegal drugs is a criminal activity. Statistics from the Bureau of Justice Statistics (BJS) highlight the connection between drug use and other crimes. According to the BJS, 83 percent of inmates in state and federal prisons in 1997 used at least one illegal drug at some time in their lives. The most frequently used illegal drugs among inmates were marijuana (77 percent of inmates reported using it), cocaine and **crack** (49 percent), **hallucinogens** (29 percent), **stimulants** (28 percent), and **opiates** and **depressants** (24 percent each).

Law enforcement officials report that a majority of all crimes are committed under the influence of drugs or alcohol. The BJS found that 55 percent of jail inmates in 1996 reported using illegal drugs in the month before their arrest. The most commonly used illegal drugs by inmates were marijuana (used by 37 percent of inmates), cocaine and crack (a combined 24 percent), and stimulants (10 percent). A BJS survey of victims of violent crime showed that 29 percent believed that their attacker was using either drugs or alcohol (or both) at the time of the offense.

Some drug-related crimes are committed to acquire money to purchase drugs. The BJS 1996 Profile of Jail Inmates found that 24 percent of property crimes were motivated by a need to purchase drugs.

In contrast, only about 14 percent of property crime offenses in 1989 were perpetrated to acquire drug money. The BJS also reported that, in 1997, 19 percent of all inmates in state prisons and 16 percent of those in federal prison said they committed their current offenses to obtain money for drugs.

More worrisome is the number of violent crimes committed by drug users. According to the BJS, over 14,000 drug-related homicides occurred in 2002, a significant decline from the peak year of 1993, when over 23,000 drug-related homicides occurred. However, in 2002 drug-related homicides represented 4.7 percent of all homicides, the highest proportion since 1998.

Homicide often involves teens. The Centers for Disease Control and Prevention (CDC) reports that homicide is the second-leading cause of death among 10- to 19-year-olds. According to the CDC, in 1998 there were 2,570 homicide deaths within that age group, with male teens murdered at four times the rate of females. Teens are not only victims of homicide but also perpetrators. In 1999, 1,763 teens under the age of 18 were arrested for homicide, accounting for roughly 10 percent of all murders in the United States.

One of the principal factors contributing to teen homicide is the number of teens carrying handguns or other weapons. The CDC reported in the June 2000 *Morbidity and Mortality Weekly Report* that almost 5 percent of teens in grades nine to 12 said they had carried a gun during the previous month. When all weapons were considered, approximately 17 percent of teens in the same grades reported carrying a gun, knife, or club to school during the previous month. The presence of so many firearms or other weapons increases the potential for violent behavior among teens. The CDC's Youth Risk Behavior Surveillance System from 1999 reported that 35.7 percent of students said they were involved in a fight the previous year.

TEENS SPEAK

I'm Worried about Kids Carrying Weapons to School

My name is Robert, and I'm scared for my safety because some kids at school are in gangs or dealing drugs. Just last week a guy got caught bringing a gun to school. He said that a gang member selling marijuana in the parking lot threatened him. The gang member flashed a knife at him and told him he better shut up or he'd be sorry. The next day he brought the gun. Nothing happened this time, but next time someone might get hurt or killed—even someone who just happened to be in the wrong place at the wrong time.

I've even thought about bringing a weapon to school myself. I'm not big and sometimes I get hassled by gang members or guys who just want to show how tough they are. I think that maybe if I had a knife or a gun they wouldn't mess with me. Then I realize how stupid it would be to take a weapon to school. I could end up killing someone or getting killed myself. Even if I never used it, if I got caught with it I'd get expelled like that guy last week. It's not worth the trouble or the risk.

Domestic violence and gang activity

Although no studies have found evidence that alcohol or drug use is directly responsible for domestic violence, many have shown some relationship between the two. In 1997, the National Center of Addiction and Substance Abuse at Columbia University interviewed over 900 child-welfare professionals about their experiences with drugs, alcohol, and domestic violence. Eighty percent of those surveyed said that substance abuse plays a role in most cases of child abuse, and 40 percent said that drugs and alcohol are involved in over 75 percent of child abuse cases. Alcohol is the drug most often associated with domestic violence. In a 1984 study of 1,500 abused wives in Philadelphia, 55 percent said their husbands became abusive after drinking alcohol.

One form of teen criminal behavior that has grown substantially since the 1980s has been gang activity. An epidemic of crack cocaine use led to an increase in the number of teens recruited by gangs to sell the drug. In their 1997 National Youth Gang Survey, the Office of Juvenile Justice and Delinquency Prevention (OJJDP) reported that approximately 33 percent of all teen gangs in the United States are involved in drug trafficking—buying and selling illegal substances. The OJJDP also reported that 42 percent of teen gangs are involved in the smaller-scale **street sale** of drugs. The profits to be made from selling drugs can entice teens into the gang lifestyle. However, the possible negative consequences of gang activity—violence, the likelihood of going to prison, or death—far outweigh possible benefits of the money generated by drug dealing.

DRUG ABUSERS AS
VICTIMS OF VIOLENCE

Abusers of drugs and alcohol are more likely to perpetrate criminal activities. They are also more likely to be victims as well. Statistics on the number of assaults committed against individuals who were under the influence of drugs or alcohol are unavailable, simply because someone high on drugs is unlikely to go to the authorities with complaints of theft or assault. However, studies do suggest that some groups of drug users are at increased risk of being victimized.

In 1994, the *Journal of the American Medical Association* article "Homicide in New York City: Cocaine Use and Firearms" found that murder rates among female drug users were much higher than among their male counterparts. The team from Cornell University Medical Center that wrote the article studied all murders in the city between 1990 and 1991. They found that 59 percent of white female murder victims, and 72 percent of African-American female victims, had been using cocaine at the time they were murdered. By contrast, 38 percent of white men and 44 percent of African-American men murdered in that period had been using cocaine.

Female substance abusers also seem to be at greater risk for domestic violence, according to a 1989 study in the *Journal of Studies on Alcohol* titled "Spousal Violence among Alcoholic Women as Compared to a Random Household Sample." The study discovered that women who abuse substances and are the victims of domestic violence are more likely to live with men who are also substance abusers. Those women are also more likely to use physical violence to retaliate for being battered, increasing their risk of suffering serious injury during a battering episode.

THE ILLEGAL DRUG TRADE AND ITS VICTIMS

One need not steal, commit assault, or kill to commit a drug-related crime. Possessing and selling drugs are crimes in their own right, crimes that claim a significant number of victims. In 2002, more than

1.5 million Americans were arrested on drug violations, of which 186,200 were juveniles.

Q & A

Question: What percentage of all drug arrests involve juvenile offenders?

Answer: According to the Bureau of Justice Statistics, 186,200 juveniles were arrested for drug violations in 2000, representing 12.1 percent of all drug arrests. This represents a significant increase since 1990, when juveniles made up only 7.4 percent of drug arrests.

The number of drug arrests as a percentage of all arrests has risen dramatically since the early-to-mid-1960s. At that time, drug violations accounted for only about one percent of all arrests in the United States. By 1990, that number increased tenfold. By contrast, the percentage of arrests for violent crimes remained almost unchanged over the same period. The percentage of alcohol-related arrests declined from more than 40 percent in the early 1960s to just over 20 percent in 1990.

According to the Drug Enforcement Agency (DEA), the market for illegal drugs in the United States is one of the most profitable in the world. As a result, it attracts the most ruthless, sophisticated, and aggressive drug traffickers in the world. Some of the most violent of these criminal groups operate out of South America; specifically, out of Columbia. Their primary drugs are cocaine and heroin, and their primary target is the affluent United States. Israeli, Russian, and Western European traffickers are heavily involved in distributing the drug ecstasy in the United States. Domestic drug traffickers also cultivate, produce, manufacture, and distribute illegal drugs. These larger groups involved in the drug trade are known as drug cartels.

Cartels are groups that control the production and distribution of drugs. They supply the individuals and street gangs involved in trafficking drugs. The cartels sell to gang leaders, who in turn recruit gang members to sell the drugs on the street. Thus, most of the gang crime associated with drug dealing ultimately can be traced back to drug cartels. Of course, in some sense, cartels play some part in most drug-related crime—both violent and property crime. Their activities fuel the flow of drugs that are related to such crimes in the United States.

Fact Or Fiction?

The three leading causes of death for teens are declining.

Fact: The rates for teen homicide, suicide, and fatal motor vehicle crashes have all declined over the past few years. Nonfatal firearm injuries from crime also declined. These reductions can be attributed to a number of factors, but an emphasis on prevention appears to have paid off. Regardless of these reductions, according to the Office of Juvenile Justice and Delinquency Prevention, teens in 1999 still accounted for 16 percent of all violent crime arrests, including 14 percent of aggravated assault arrests, 17 percent of forcible rape arrests, and 24 percent of weapons arrests.

See also: Families, Communities, and Drug Abuse; Gangs and Drugs; Homicide; Illegal Drugs, Common; Law on Drugs, The

FURTHER READING

Adint, Victor. *Drugs and Crime.* New York: Rosen Publishing Group, 1994.

Benson, Bruce L. and David W. Rasmussen. *Illegal Drugs and Crime.* Oakland, CA: Liberty Tree Network, 1996.

Martin, John M. and Anne T. Romano. *Multinational Crime: Terrorism, Espionage, Drug and Arms Trafficking.* Thousand Oaks, CA: Sage Publishing, 1992.

■ DRUGS AND DEVELOPMENT

All drugs produce short-term effects that can be harmful to the physical, emotional, and mental well-being of the user. For example, **marijuana** has been shown to impair the user's ability to concentrate and perform simple tasks using large and small muscle groups. Most drugs also have serious long-term effects on the user's behavior, physical health, and mental development. The destructive effects of substance abuse can begin even before birth if a woman uses drugs during pregnancy. Individuals who use drugs during childhood and adolescence are at substantial risk of stunted physical, emotional, or mental development. Many factors other than drug use (poverty, for example) can contribute to unhealthy development in an individual. However, drug abuse frequently compounds the negative effects of other unhealthy developmental influences in an individual's environment.

PREGNANCY AND DRUGS

Because pregnant women share blood and other vital nutrients with their unborn children, any substance consumed by the mother is passed along to the child. Mothers who eat a healthful diet during pregnancy typically bear stronger, healthier children than those who do not. Similarly, if a mother abuses drugs during pregnancy, her unborn child will receive the drug and suffer from the effects of that drug. Medical studies have demonstrated that drug use during pregnancy can have serious negative effects on the development of the exposed child. In fact, the vast majority of all studies of drugs on child development have focused on the prenatal (before birth) use of drugs by pregnant women.

COCAINE AND CRACK COCAINE

In recent years **cocaine** and crack cocaine have been among the drugs subjected to the most scientific research regarding their effects on development. The dramatic increase in the use of crack since the 1980s has prompted much of the interest in the developmental effects of cocaine use. One by-product of the so-called crack epidemic was an intense interest in developmental difficulties exhibited by infants whose mothers used crack during pregnancy. In the 1990s, both the popular and scientific press ran a variety of stories about the problem of "crack babies." While later research called into question some of the initial conclusions about the health effects of prenatal exposure to crack, it is clear that both crack and powder cocaine have profound negative effects on development.

Cognitive development

In 2002, researchers from Case Western Reserve University School of Medicine, MetroHealth Medical Center, and University Hospitals of Cleveland published an extensive study in the *Journal of the American Medical Association* titled "Cognitive and Motor Outcomes of Cocaine-Exposed Infants." The researchers compared the cognitive (mental) and motor development (the use of large and small muscle groups) of 415 infants who were exposed to cocaine before birth to nonexposed infants. The study, which followed the infants from birth until age two, found that prenatal cocaine exposure affects a child's cognitive development but not motor development.

According to the study, cocaine-exposed infants were more likely to be born prematurely, weigh less at birth, and have smaller heads and bodies than nonexposed infants. The researchers also found that at age two cocaine-exposed infants had nearly five times the rate of mental retardation as the general population. In addition, 37.6 percent of the cocaine-exposed children showed "mild" developmental retardation that required some type of educational intervention, as compared with 20.9 percent in the nonexposed group. The study suggests that these children are likely to have learning problems well into childhood and will probably need special educational services once they enter school.

According to a 1999 study that appeared in the journal *Clinics in Perinatology* titled "Prenatal Drug Exposure and Child Outcomes," researchers have found other evidence of negative cognitive effects caused by cocaine exposure. The study reported that cocaine affects the development of brain regions that regulate attention, arousal, and reaction to stress. Cocaine-exposed children scored lower than non-exposed children on tests measuring alertness, attention, and intelligence. Although the effects were not dramatic, the researchers found that they last through early childhood. As a result of the study, they suggest that cocaine-exposed children will have more trouble focusing their attention, remaining alert, and processing information than nonexposed children.

Other research has confirmed that cocaine negatively impacts attention and alertness into childhood. A 1998 study from the *Annals of the New York Academy of Sciences* titled "Regulation of Arousal and Attention in Preschool Children Exposed to Cocaine Prenatally" suggests that cocaine affects a child's ability to pay attention, which can seriously impact learning and memory. The article noted that cocaine-exposed children appear to require more stimulation to increase their levels of arousal and attention. At the same time, however, they are emotionally less able to control higher states of arousal than nonexposed children.

In 2000, an article in the journal *Pediatrics* titled "Adverse Effects of Fetal Cocaine Exposure on Neonatal Auditory Information

Processing" found that infants exposed to cocaine perform much more poorly than nonexposed infants on a test that identifies children at risk of delayed cognitive development. Infants who fare poorly on the test may be at greater risk for impaired attention and language abilities in later childhood.

Motor and physical development

Cocaine exposure can affect not only a child's cognitive development but also his or her motor development. Research conducted at Case Western Reserve University in Cleveland has shown links between prenatal cocaine exposure and decreased motor development in children at age two. According to the 1999 study "Motor Development of Cocaine-Exposed Children at Age Two Years," exposed children performed significantly poorer than nonexposed children on tests of both fine and gross motor development. The study concluded that "the lag in development extends beyond the neonatal period (the period immediately following birth) in exposed children."

Researchers had previously found that cocaine-exposed children who had problems in motor development at the age of four months continued to lag behind other children as late as the age of two years. Studies of the same children at age four suggest that cocaine-related problems with fine motor development last into early childhood. As the study noted, it is difficult for a child to control a pencil without properly developed motor skills. Such difficulties can negatively impact early school performance.

Q & A

Question: What is fetal alcohol syndrome?

Answer: Fetal alcohol syndrome (FAS) is a developmental condition caused by prenatal exposure to alcohol. It is marked by physical, mental, and behavioral problems that are apparent immediately after birth. Babies with FAS show physical symptoms such as small heads, narrow eye slits, a flat and long upper lip, flattened nose, and underdeveloped and central face area. FAS babies usually have a low birth weight and are small for their age. Other physical problems linked to FAS include problems with blood circulation, heart murmurs, kidney trouble, respiratory difficulty, hernias, and shortened fingers. These infants also show delayed motor development that, in many cases, never becomes normal. A significant number of FAS children also suffer from impaired vision and/or hearing that can affect learning ability.

These children also suffer cognitive impairments, including difficulty comprehending language and processing and storing information. Children with FAS typically have IQ scores ranging from normal to severely mentally retarded, with a mean score of 65 (100 is considered average). These scores do not appear to improve over time. Clearly, FAS is a serious disorder that should caution all women against drinking during pregnancy.

HEROIN AND OTHER OPIATES

Heroin, which is produced from the Asian poppy plant, is part of a class of drugs known as **opiates.** Opiates, which also include opium and morphine, are among the most powerful illicit drugs. They produce profound physical and mental effects, including extreme drowsiness and a sense of **euphoria.** Prenatal exposure to opiates can have negative consequences for mental and physical development.

Cognitive development

According to researcher Karol Kaltenbach of the National Institute on Drug Abuse (NIDA), most of the research into the effects of opiates on infants comes from several long-range studies conducted in the 1970s and 1980s. A number of these studies compared cognitive development in opiate-exposed children with nonexposed children and found that opiate-exposed children did not perform as well on several tests of cognitive development: the acquisition of skills necessary to think, reason, and solve problems. A 1988 article in the *Annals of the New York Academy of Sciences* titled "Drug-Addicted Mothers, Their Infants, and SIDS" reported that opiate-exposed infants had lower scores on the Bayley Mental Development Index at 12 and 18 months of age than nonexposed infants. According to a 1979 study in the journal *Pediatrics* titled "The Development of Preschool Children of Heroin-Addicted Mothers," heroin-exposed children also performed more poorly than nonexposed children on the General Cognitive Index.

Despite these findings, a number of other studies have found little or no differences in cognitive development among opiate-exposed children. According to Kaltenbach, later researchers found that environmental factors such as poverty or continued drug use by the mother contributed significantly to the cognitive delays experienced by heroin-exposed children.

Motor and physical development

A larger body of evidence suggests that heroin and other opiates negatively impact motor development. A 1976 study in the journal *Pediatrics* titled "Behavioral Concomitants of Prenatal Addiction to Narcotics" found that scores of opiate-exposed children on the Motor Development Index declined as the children grew older. According to the 1982 study "Children of Methadone-Maintained Mothers: Follow-up to 18 Months of Age," heroin-exposed infants performed about the same as nonexposed infants on the Motor Development Index (MDI) at six months of age but substantially worse at 12 and 18 months. A 1989 study titled "Developmental Consequences to Prenatal Exposure to Methadone" found that heroin-exposed infants scored lower on the MDI and had poorer motor coordination than nonexposed infants.

Researchers have also noted a pattern of behavior among heroin-exposed infants known as neonatal abstinence. This condition is marked by irritability, intestinal distress, respiratory problems, and other symptoms such as sneezing, discoloration of the skin, and fever. Such infants may suck frantically on their hands or thumbs and may have trouble breast-feeding because of an uncoordinated sucking reflex. Infants undergoing neonatal abstinence can develop tremors and become extremely irritable. Neonatal abstinence is a form of **withdrawal** experienced by infants who have been exposed to heroin. If the condition is treated immediately it typically has no long-term negative effects.

MARIJUANA

Although the physical and cognitive effects of **marijuana** are less intense than those of cocaine or heroin, marijuana still presents a number of developmental risks. Because marijuana is one of the drugs most widely used by adolescents, researchers have more data about the effects of marijuana on development in later childhood and adolescence than they do about many other drugs.

Cognitive development

Long-term studies have revealed subtle cognitive deficits in the children of mothers who smoked marijuana during pregnancy. A 1991 study in the journal *Clinical Perinatology* titled "Animal Models of Opiate, Cocaine, and Cannabis Use" suggested that marijuana-exposed infants were more likely to experience learning and memory impairment but did not find these effects to be lasting.

In 2001, the American Academy of Pediatrics (AAP) put marijuana on its list of drugs that adversely affect infants during breast-feeding. According to the AAP, the active ingredient in marijuana, THC, can be stored in a mother's tissues for several weeks or months and accumulates with continued use. Thomas Hale, author of the book *Medications and Mother's Milk*, reports that breast milk produced by chronic, heavy marijuana users shows extremely high concentrations of THC. Marijuana taken into the body through breast-feeding can cause sleepiness in the baby, which may lead to slow weight gain and possibly slow overall development. The study also found that babies whose mothers smoke marijuana regularly have a higher risk of dying from Sudden Infant Death Syndrome, or SIDS.

Much research has been devoted to the cognitive and behavioral effects of marijuana on adolescents and adults. Many of the effects described earlier involved the performance of a complex combination of cognitive and motor skills. A 1995 study by the Australian government titled "The Health and Psychological Consequences of Cannabis Use" found that heavy marijuana use may produce subtle cognitive impairment. Marijuana appears to have its greatest effect on short-term memory. According to a 1993 article titled "Chronic Marihuana Smoking and Short-term Memory Impairment," marijuana use in adolescents may also result in long-term memory impairment. Evidence from a 1996 study in the *Journal of the American Medical Association* titled "The Residual Cognitive Effects of Heavy Marijuana Use in College Students" suggests that chronic marijuana use over many years may cause subtle reductions in attention as well as in the ability to organize and make sense of complex information. According to a 1995 article titled "The Health and Psychological Consequences of Cannabis Use," part of the National Drug Strategy Monograph Series, there may be a modest relationship between marijuana use in adolescence and poor academic performance.

Motor and physical development
Aside from its cognitive effects, marijuana has been linked to some impairment of motor functions and a range of long-term health problems. A 1990 study published in the journal *Neurotoxicology and*

Teratology titled "Maternal Marijuana Use During Lactation and Infant Development at One Year" found that infants exposed to marijuana through their mother's milk during the first month of life showed decreased motor development at one year of age.

Several studies have detailed the risk of developing cancer as a result of smoking marijuana. According to a 1999 article in the journal *Cancer Epidemiology* titled "Marijuana Use and Increased Risk of Squamous Cell Carcinoma of the Head and Neck," smoking marijuana increases the likelihood of developing cancer of the head or neck. The study, which compared 173 cancer patients and 176 healthy individuals, suggested that marijuana smoking doubled the risk of developing these cancers. The same study reported that marijuana use may also promote cancer of the lungs and other parts of the respiratory tract. A 1981 report from the *Annals of the New York Academy of Sciences* titled "Adverse Effects of Marijuana: Selected Issues" found that marijuana may also accelerate the changes in cells that produce cancer.

Some evidence suggests that smoking marijuana may result in long-term impairment of the immune system, which is responsible for fighting infections. A 1997 study from the Center for Substance Abuse Prevention titled "Effects of Marijuana on the Lung and Its Immune Defenses" reported that marijuana may suppress the activity of a variety of immune cells that fight disease. The article cited studies that found that the lungs of habitual marijuana smokers showed a reduced ability to kill fungal and bacterial organisms as well as tumor cells. These findings suggest that marijuana can have significant negative effects on the body's natural defenses, which could have potentially serious health consequences for users with other immune system problems arising from **AIDS**, cancer, or an organ transplant.

Somewhat surprisingly, no conclusive evidence links marijuana with long-term developmental problems with lung function and respiratory health. For example, a 1987 article in the *British Medical Journal* titled "Respiratory Effects of Non-Tobacco Cigarettes" reported that smoking an average of one marijuana cigarette per day was linked to significant impairment in small airways in the lungs. The authors of the study concluded that regular marijuana smoking was a risk factor for the development of chronic obstructive pulmonary disease (COPD), which is marked by a disabling shortness of breath. In contrast, a 1987 study published in the *American Journal of Respiratory and Critical Care Medicine* titled "Heavy Habitual Marijuana Smoking Does Not Cause an Accelerated Decline in FEV1 with Age: A Longitudinal

Study" found no impairment in the function of small airways in association with regular use of marijuana (three cigarettes per day). These mixed findings leave open the question as to whether regular smoking of marijuana alone can lead to COPD.

TEENS SPEAK

I used to think that doing drugs was just a personal choice and that the person using them was the only one who could get hurt. I found out differently, though, when my sister's baby was born.

My sister Katie experimented with drugs when she was younger. When she got married, she stopped doing some of the drugs she had tried in college. The one drug she still did, however, was methamphetamine. Katy worked long hours at her job, and she was often in her office until past midnight. Sometimes she'd work until six o'clock or so, then come home for dinner and head right back to the office. A lot of the time she had trouble staying alert and concentrating, so she took methamphetamine to give her energy and fight sleepiness. I was really worried about her using the drug, but she said she could handle it and that it wasn't a problem for her.

I began to worry even more after she got pregnant. I had heard in health class that almost any drug can cause problems for an unborn child, but that cocaine and methamphetamine were supposed to be really dangerous. I tried to get her to stop because of what she might do to her baby. For three months I got nowhere with her, but finally after her husband and some friends put pressure on her, she agreed to stop. Because of the pregnancy she wasn't working full-time, so she didn't need to stay up so late anymore.

I thought we stopped her in time, but when her baby was born it was five weeks early and very small and weak. The baby trembled, twitched, and cried, and it looked very sickly. For weeks I was afraid the baby would die. Luckily my sister was in a hospital where the doctors and nurses were able to take care of her child. The baby is now six months old, and although he is still smaller and weaker than other babies, he is alive and getting healthier. It just goes to show that drugs can hurt other people even more than the person who uses them, especially when the other person is a baby.

METHAMPHETAMINE

Although cocaine, opiates, and marijuana have been the drugs most extensively studied for effects on development, research has also shed light on the negative developmental impact of **methamphetamine**. The drug has been found to impair infant development as well as cognitive and emotional development in later life.

Prenatal effects

Studies of methamphetamine use by pregnant women have revealed several areas of physical and mental impairment in methamphetamine-exposed infants. According to a 2003 study published in the *Journal of Developmental and Behavioral Pediatrics* titled "Effects of Prenatal Methamphetamine Exposure on Fetal Growth and Drug Withdrawal Symptoms in Infants Born at Term," methamphetamine use during pregnancy was associated with delayed growth during early infancy. In addition, the group of methamphetamine-exposed infants observed in the study contained a significantly higher percentage of small-for-age infants than the nonexposed group. These findings suggest that methamphetamine use can lead to reduced growth during infancy.

Michael Sherman, chief of neonatology at the University of California–Davis Medical Center has found evidence of other negative effects from prenatal methamphetamine use. These include damage to the brain and spinal cord, malformation of the kidneys, problems with the development of the intestines, and skeletal abnormalities. Sherman also describes a condition called gastroschesis, in which the infant develops a hole in the abdominal wall and its intestines are outside the body. According to Sherman, this birth defect is common in mothers who abuse methamphetamine during pregnancy. Other problems noted in methamphetamine-exposed infants include cerebral palsy, seizures, paralysis, irritability, attention problems, hyperactivity, and delayed development.

Effects on later development

Adolescents who use methamphetamine expose themselves to the risk of developing severe behavioral and physical problems into adulthood. According to NIDA, chronic methamphetamine use can lead to violent behavior, anxiety, confusion, insomnia, **paranoia**, **hallucinations**, **delusions**, and mood disturbances. Paranoia caused by chronic methamphetamine use can result in homicidal and suicidal thoughts. Long-term use can cause increased blood pressure and significantly increase the chances of suffering a stroke. Other long-term physical effects include respiratory problems, irregular heartbeat, and extreme **anorexia**.

NIDA also reports several severe long-term effects on brain development in adulthood. For example, methamphetamine appears to damage brain cells in a way that can result in symptoms similar to those of Parkinson's disease, a disorder marked by extreme, uncontrollable trembling of the limbs. According to NIDA, high doses of methamphetamine can also damage nerve cell endings, and the ability of these cells to recover appears to be limited.

Fact Or Fiction?

Prenatal exposure to ecstasy causes developmental problems in infants.

Fact: The evidence for developmental problems due to use of ecstasy during pregnancy is mixed. A long-term study of infants born to mothers in Great Britain who used methylenedioxymethamphetamine (ecstasy) during pregnancy found some increased risk of birth defects. Patricia R. McElhatton and colleagues of the National Teratology Information Service in Newcastle upon Tyne, United Kingdom, studied 136 pregnancies that occurred between 1989 and 1998. Among the women studied, 74 had taken ecstasy alone, and the other 62 took a combination of ecstasy and another drug. The study found that 15.4 percent of the infants had birth defects, compared with an expected rate of 2 to 3 percent. McElhatton said that it is unclear whether the birth defects resulted from the combined effects of mixing drugs or whether they were caused by ecstasy alone. Although she cautioned that the results do not prove a direct link between ecstasy and birth defects, they suggested that either ecstasy or amphetamines played some role.

THE IMPACT OF DRUG USE

There can be no question that many illegal drugs have a profoundly negative impact on both early and later development. Pregnant mothers who abuse drugs should be aware that they are sharing these substances with their unborn children, who are far less prepared to suffer the effects. Substance abuse that occurs during pregnancy can be the start of lifelong developmental problems for an exposed child, and continued abuse as an adolescent can seriously impair the quality of later life.

See also: Crack Cocaine; Dependence and Addiction; Drugs and Criminal Activity; Illegal Drugs, Common; Law on Drugs, The; Morbidity and Mortality

FURTHER READING

Corser, Kira and Frances Paine Adler. *When the Bough Breaks: Pregnancy and the Legacy of Addiction.* Portland, OR: New Sage Press, 1993.

Inciardi, James A., Hilary L. Surratt, and Christine A. Saum. *Cocaine-Exposed Infants: Social, Legal, and Public Health Issues.* Thousand Oaks, CA: Sage Publications, 1997.

Thomas, Janey Y. *Educating Drug-Exposed Children: The Aftermath of the Crack-Baby Crisis.* London, UK: Fallmer Press, 2004.

■ DRUGS AND DISEASE

A condition that impairs normal physical or psychological functioning. One of the least-appreciated drawbacks to using drugs is the possibility of developing mental disorders or contracting a serious disease such as **hepatitis** (an infectious disease that can cause serious liver damage) or **HIV/AIDS.** HIV is a virus that attacks the body's immune system and causes AIDS, a medical condition in which the body's immune system is so weakened that even mild infections can cause serious illness or death. Knowing about the health risks associated with drugs can help you realize just how dangerous drug use can be.

DRUG PSYCHOSIS

Psychosis is a severe mental disorder marked by a loss of contact with reality. Taking drugs can produce a condition called **drug psychosis**

that generates symptoms similar to those found in other forms of psychosis. Common symptoms include **hallucinations** (seeing, hearing, and smelling things that are not there) and **delusions** (false beliefs held even in the face of contrary evidence). Drug-induced psychosis can occur during the drug experience, while coming down off the drug, or when withdrawing from the drug. Since different drugs exit the body at varying times during the **withdrawal** period, an episode of drug-induced psychosis may start weeks after last taking a drug.

Typically, drugs do not **trigger** (set off) a psychotic episode unless a mental illness is present. Although a family or personal history of psychotic illness increases the risk of drug psychosis, it is not necessary to trigger a drug-induced psychotic episode. Stress or drugs like **amphetamines** (synthetically produced stimulants that improve alertness and elevate mood), **LSD** (a synthetic hallucinogen), **ecstasy** (a synthetically produced substance that produce a wide range of drug effects) and **marijuana** (an illicit drug derived from hemp that alters mood and distorts the senses) have been known to trigger an episode in an otherwise healthy person. Using multiple drugs all at once can also increase the chances of drug psychosis.

The onset and length of an episode can vary depending on the drug. A single dose of cocaine may produce a psychotic episode in a matter of minutes, while other substances may take longer. Marijuana may produce drug psychosis for a few days, but with amphetamines or **cocaine** (an addictive drug, derived from the coca plant, that increases energy and alertness), the drug induced psychosis can last for weeks, even after quitting the drug. Most people recover from drug-induced psychosis with treatment and by quitting the drugs. In some cases, however, **tranquilizers** (depressants that relieve anxiety) may be needed to reduce the likelihood of suicidal or aggressive behavior.

DEPRESSION

Depression is a mental disorder caused by a chemical imbalance in the brain, characterized by feelings of profound sadness, hopeless, and worthlessness. Depression and drug use have a unique relationship. Some people may begin using illegal drugs or alcohol or increase their use of these substances in response to depression. In turn, the use of alcohol and drugs can deepen the depression. That cycle, in which drug use and depression reinforce one another, is dangerous.

Illegal drugs and alcohol are especially dangerous when taken in addition to antidepressant medication. **Antidepressants** work by subtly altering the brain's chemistry to maintain normal mental functioning. Alcohol and illegal drugs can interfere with this process, making the antidepressant less effective. In addition, drugs and alcohol can increase the side effects associated with many antidepressants, such as sleep disruption, headaches, nausea, agitation, and anxiety. As with any depression, suicide is always a concern, especially when drugs and alcohol are being abused.

HIV/AIDS

The Centers for Disease Control and Prevention (CDC) reports that HIV/AIDS was the fifth-leading cause of death for Americans between the ages of 25 and 44 in 1999 and the leading cause among African-American men in that age group since 1991. HIV—the virus that causes AIDS, a serious and often fatal disease of the immune system transmitted through blood products—has a long incubation period during which the virus is present but dormant with no outward symptoms. As a result, many of those in the 25–44 age group were infected in their teens. Philip Rosenberg and Robert J. Biggar of the National Cancer Institute estimate that at least one-half of all HIV infections in the United States are among people under the age of 25. In 2000, 1,688 people between the ages of 13 and 24 were diagnosed with AIDS, bringing the total number of recorded cases of AIDS in this age group to 31,293 since the CDC began keeping records in the 1980s.

Among young men ages 13–24, 10 percent of all AIDS cases reported in 2000 were **injection drug** users and 9 percent were among young men infected heterosexually. Injection drugs are drugs that are injected into the veins or muscles of the user with a needle. Among young women of the same age, 11 percent of all AIDS cases reported were acquired through injection drug use. In 2000, drug injection led to at least 6 percent of HIV diagnoses reported among those ages 13–24.

Fact Or Fiction?

The greatest risk for teens of acquiring HIV/AIDS is through injection drug use.

Fact: Fifty percent of all HIV/AIDS diagnoses in teenagers are acquired through sexual transmission, making unprotected sexual behavior the greatest HIV/AIDS risk for teens. Many teens report using alcohol or drugs when they have sex, which can negatively impact the use of protection.

Data from the CDC suggests that drug injection led to at least six percent of HIV diagnoses reported among those between the ages of 13 and 24 in 2000. Although injection drug use among teens is low, other drug and alcohol use can diminish sexual inhibitions and cloud one's judgment thus creating the potential for unprotected intercourse. Unprotected sexual intercourse provides the greatest risk of HIV infection for teens, to say nothing of the increased risk of sexually transmitted viruses.

Drug use can be particularly dangerous for sexually active youth because it can diminish sexual inhibitions and cloud one's judgment. These conditions create the potential for unprotected sexual intercourse, which provides the greatest risk of not only HIV infection but also **sexually transmitted diseases** such as syphilis and gonorrhea.

HEPATITIS

Hepatitis is an inflammation of the liver caused by an infection, drugs, toxins, or parasites. The disease is characterized by an enlarged liver, jaundice, diminished appetite, nausea, and abdominal pain. There are several different forms of the disease. The most common is hepatitis A virus (HAV). Although all forms attack the liver to some extent, hepatitis B and C, which can cause liver cancer, are of special concern because they are the most deadly varieties.

HAV is usually spread from person to person by contaminated food or water and personal contact. HAV has no long-term effects, but about 15 percent of people infected have prolonged or recurring symptoms over a six- to nine-month period. The greatest risk of acquiring HAV is through contact with infected persons. The best protection against hepatitis is a vaccine.

Q & A

Question: What kinds of activities increase the chances of acquiring an infectious disease?

Answer: The following behaviors increase the risk of contracting an infectious disease:

- Injecting drugs with dirty or used needles
- Sharing needles or other paraphernalia associated with injection drugs

- Sharing razors, toothbrushes, or other personal grooming items with an injection drug user
- Having unprotected sex
- Getting tattoos or body piercings with unsterilized equipment

Hepatitis B (HVB) may be transmitted through sexual intercourse and through contaminated blood or needles. HVB has declined in recent years, primarily because of the widespread availability of a vaccine. The number of new infections has dropped from an average of 260,000 per year in the 1980s to about 78,000 in 2001. Although the highest rate of disease occurs among 20- to 49-year-olds, the most significant reduction has been among children and teens. The symptoms are very similar to those associated with HAV with the exception of joint pain. However, roughly 30 percent of those infected with HVB have no symptoms at all. Children are less likely to show symptoms than adults. If HVB is not treated, the liver can develop chronic infection. Death from chronic liver disease occurs in about 15–25 percent of those infected.

HVB transmission occurs when blood or other body fluids from an infected person enters the body of someone who is not immune. There are three primary modes of transmission: having sex with an infected person without using protection; using or being stuck with an infected needle; and being born to an infected mother.

HVB can be prevented if these rules are followed:

- Don't use injection drugs.
- Always use protection if engaging in sex.
- Never share needles.

Hepatitis C (HVC) is spread primarily by injection drug use. The number of new infections per year has declined from an average of 240,000 in the 1980s to about 25,000 in 2001. Roughly 4 million Americans have been infected with HCV, with 2.7 million chronically infected. Chronic infection occurs in 75–85 percent of those infected. The rate of chronic infection is so high because over 75 percent of those infected have no symptoms. Approximately 70 percent of those infected will acquire chronic liver disease, and a small proportion of them will suffer liver damage so severe they will require a liver transplant. The

CDC estimates that illicit injection drug use causes 60 percent of all new cases of HCV and is also a primary factor in HVB infection.

Transmission of HCV is very similar to HVB and occurs when blood or body fluids from an infected person enters the body of a person who is not infected. To prevent infection follow rules similar to those outlined for avoiding HBV. The major difference between HBV and HCV is that no vaccine exists to prevent HCV, although treatment can eliminate the virus in 50 percent of those infected.

Hepatitis D and E are less common and less dangerous viruses than the A, B, and C strains. Hepatitis D is a virus that is found in the blood of persons infected with HVB, and it needs that virus to exist. Hepatitis E, a virus transmitted in much the same way as HAV, does not often occur in the United States.

Avoiding risky behaviors such as drug use and unprotected sex is the only effective way to prevent the spread of diseases such as HIV/AIDS and hepatitis. The effects of injection drugs such as heroin are dangerous enough, but the possibility of contracting a serious disease from a contaminated needle makes them particularly lethal. Don't be fooled into believing that drugs other than injection drugs are somehow safe. Any drug can impair judgment and increase the chances of taking a deadly risk that no one would even consider when sober.

See also: Depression and Drugs; Drugs and Drinking; Injection Drugs; Sexual Behavior and Drug Abuse

FURTHER READING

Evans, C. *Illicit Drug Use and HIV Infection.* Washington, DC: American Public Health Association, 1989.

Hagan, Elizabeth and Joan Gormley. *HIV/AIDS and the Drug Culture: Shattered Lives.* Binghamton, NY: The Haworth Press, 1998.

Palfreeman, Adrian, Michael Youle, and Charles F. Farthing. *Drugs in HIV and AIDS*, 2nd ed. Hoboken, NJ: John Wiley and Sons, 1998.

Turkington, Carol. *Hepatitis C: The Silent Epidemic.* Chicago: Contemporary Books, 1998.

■ DRUGS AND DRINKING

Alcohol is by far the most commonly used drug among teens. According to the National Institute on Drug Abuse, in 2003 almost half of all eighth graders, two-thirds of 10th graders, and over three-quarters of 12th graders had used alcohol. These figures are particularly troubling, because alcohol has been identified as a gateway drug—a substance whose use may lead to the abuse of other drugs. Although the relationship between teen alcohol use and illegal drugs is unclear, there seems to be a link between the two.

Fact Or Fiction?

Teenage alcohol use continues to rise.

Fact: Alcohol use among teens is declining. According to the Centers for Disease Control and Prevention, the rates for teen alcohol use between 2001 and 2003 dropped significantly in the categories of past-year and past-month use. For example, the percentage of high school students who reported having at least one drink of alcohol within the previous 30 days dropped from 47.1 percent in 2001 to 44.9 percent in 2003. In the same time period, fewer eighth and 10th graders reported ever having ever been drunk or having been drunk in the last year.

Alcohol and drug use are also linked closely to a number of mental and physical problems, including depression. Alcohol and drugs can trigger depression, and the sadness and despair associated with depression can in turn trigger alcohol and drug use. Depression, alcohol, and drugs don't mix. The qualities of alcohol and barbiturates—drugs that slow down the functions of the central nervous system—are of special concern because these drugs can intensify the feelings of sadness or worthlessness that accompany depression. Depending on the severity of the depression, the use of alcohol and drugs may create a situation that could lead to a suicide attempt. Because suicide is one of the leading killers of teens, this relationship should not be taken too lightly.

Q & A

Question: How likely is a teen to ride with someone who has been drinking?

Answer: Research from the Centers for Disease Control and Prevention (Youth Risk Behavior Surveillance System, 1999) has shown that about one-third of teenagers reported riding with someone who had been drinking within the last 30 days. Compounding that risk is another statistic: Approximately 16 percent of teens reported rarely or never wearing a seat belt.

The role of alcohol and drugs in crime is one of the most well-documented relationships in criminal justice. In 2002 the Bureau of Justice Statistics reported that 29 percent of victims of violent crime said their attacker was under the influence of drugs or alcohol. According to a 1994 report by the National Institute of Justice titled "Psychoactive Substances and Violence," the consumption of alcohol increases aggression, as does the consumption of **cocaine, amphetamines,** and **hallucinogens.** They all can produce violent behaviors. The report suggested that other illicit drugs such as **heroin** and **marijuana** are more closely aligned with crimes related to the sales and marketing of drugs, including disputes among drug dealers and burglary and other property crimes committed to raise money for drugs.

Gang violence, drugs, and alcohol are also a dangerous combination. The use of drugs and alcohol among teens in gangs can lead to a variety of criminal activities. Drug trafficking, turf wars, and drug deals gone bad all are situations where tensions are high. The addition of drug and alcohol in an already tense situation is a recipe for violence. Homicide among teens is one of the three leading causes of death for this group.

The effects of any illicit drug can be negatively affected by the addition of alcohol. Sometimes combining illicit drugs and alcohol will intensify the reaction caused by the drugs; at other times the mixture will produce a completely different reaction from what you expect. It is clear that mixing drugs and alcohol is very dangerous.

The questionable formulas of drugs produced in clandestine basement laboratories make mixing them with alcohol especially dangerous. **Methamphetamines, designer drugs,** and **club drugs** often contain impurities and ingredients whose reaction with alcohol can be dangerously unpredictable. The so-called **date rape drugs** can also be very dangerous when used with alcohol. These drugs are powerful **sedatives** and their use with alcohol can cause life functions to be slowed so extensively that coma and death occur.

Sexual activity among teens is closely associated with alcohol and drug use. Of the roughly 33 percent of teens who engage in sexual intercourse, about a quarter reported using drugs and alcohol the last time they had intercourse. The use of alcohol and drugs by sexually active teens may also lead to risky behaviors such as having unprotected sex, which increases the risk of sexually transmitted diseases (STDs).

Many risks are associated with alcohol and drug use. It is important for teens to think *before* they use these substances, because drugs and alcohol impair one's ability to make reasoned decisions *after* he or she takes them. And when facing the possibility of adverse drug effects, automobile accidents, or STDs, the best protection is clear thinking and good judgment.

TEENS SPEAK

I Didn't Think Drinking Was Such a Big Deal

My name is Derek, and along with my buddies on the football team, I drink beer on the weekends. We party a lot, but we figured, "Hey, at least we're not doing drugs." What we didn't realize was that alcohol is a drug that can be just as dangerous as marijuana or other illegal drugs. Sure, we'd heard that alcohol was a gateway drug that could lead to other kinds of drug use, but we thought that was just something the teachers say to scare you.

I started to question how smart drinking was when my friend Robby got stopped for a DUI (driving under the influence of alcohol). He'd only had a few beers, but he was weaving enough that a police officer pulled him over. Robby lost his license for six months, but he's lucky he wasn't in an accident.

Then last Friday, Craig, another buddy from the team, told me he had some marijuana and asked me if I wanted to smoke with him. I told him no, but I was really shocked that he would use drugs. Later I thought about alcohol being a gateway drug. I guess it isn't as ridiculous as it sounds. I'm glad I turned Craig down, but I think maybe I should talk to him about marijuana *and* alcohol. Both of them can lead to big trouble.

See also: Club and Designer Drugs; Depression and Drugs; Drugs and Criminal Activity; Gangs and Drugs; Homicide; Sexual Behavior and Drug Abuse

■ FAMILIES, COMMUNITIES, AND DRUG ABUSE

Drug abuse is the nonmedical use of a substance taken to affect one's mental processes, satisfy a dependence (the compulsive use of a drug despite harmful psychological, physical, or social consequences), or attempt suicide. Families affect drug use by the kind of messages they send about its acceptability as well as by how they react to drug abuse by family members. The surrounding community also plays a role. It may either reinforce the messages communicated within the family, or challenge and question those messages. Dealing with neighborhood influences that may lead teens to use drugs or alcohol is one of the most important challenges faced by parents today.

DRUG ABUSE AND FAMILIES

Drug abuse is often a family affair. Family attitudes, actions, and interactions have a profound influence on a teen's behavior. That influence may be positive or negative, and it can start even before birth. A 1992 study conducted by the National Institute on Drug Abuse (NIDA) found that more than 5 percent of pregnant women had used at least one illegal drug. According to NIDA, **marijuana** and **cocaine** were the drugs most often used during pregnancy.

In following up the study, researchers learned that children who had been exposed to drugs while in the womb were at greater risk for various behavior problems, including difficulty delaying gratification, handling frustration, and dealing with stress. A 1998 study by Linda Mayes of the Yale University Child Study Center found that the negative effects of cocaine use during pregnancy still affected children years later. At two years of age, children exposed to prenatal cocaine use showed more impulsive behavior and suffered more from delays in acquiring language skills than nonexposed children. Such children were also more likely to be held back a grade in school and to require special education classes.

Drugs and family violence

Physical damage to children exposed to drugs prenatally is but one of many negative effects that drugs can have on family life. Studies have also shown a strong connection between drugs, alcohol, and family violence. According to a survey of 915 child-welfare professionals sponsored by the National Center of Addiction and Substance Abuse at Columbia University, most expressed a belief that parental substance abuse produced "chaos, collapse, and calamity, leaving behind a wreckage of millions of children." In the opinion of 80 percent of the respondents, substance abuse directly causes or plays a role in most cases of child abuse. Forty percent said that drugs and alcohol were involved in over 75 percent of the child abuse cases they handle. The respondents reported that the number of cases of child abuse more than doubled between 1986 and 1997. Seventy percent of these professionals named substance abuse as one of the three leading causes for the increase.

Alcohol is the drug most often associated with domestic violence. A 1984 article in *Alcohol Treatment Quarterly* titled "Alcohol-Related Domestic Violence: Clinical Implications and Intervention Strategies" showed how close the connection is between alcohol and domestic violence. The authors studied 1,500 cases of women who sought help from abusive husbands by calling a hotline in Philadelphia. Over one-half—55 percent—said their husbands became abusive after drinking. Research has shown that children of abusive parents are at greater risk of becoming child and spouse abusers themselves. In the article "Men Who Batter: Some Personality Characteristics," the *Journal of Nervous and Mental Disease* reported in 1983 that boys who are raised by an abusive parent are more likely to abuse their spouses as adults.

Drugs and family breakup

Drug and alcohol abuse can also lead to divorce or severe family disruption. According to *Psychiatric Disorders in America: The Epidemiologic Catchment Area Study*, in 1991, alcoholics represented 24.2 percent of all Americans who had been divorced or separated more than once. By contrast, only 8.9 percent of those in intact marriages were alcoholics.

In 2000, the U.S. Conference of Mayors reported that families with children made up about 36 percent of the homeless, and that requests for emergency shelter by families increased by 17 percent between 1999 and 2000. Other studies suggest substance abuse played a significant role in these increases. In their 1991 article "Homeless and Dual Diagnosis," Robert Drake and his colleagues reported that 30–40 percent of the nation's homeless have a substance abuse problem.

In addition, the U.S. Conference of Mayors found that domestic violence was a primary cause of homelessness.

Parental attitudes and concerns

In a 2000 Gallup opinion poll, 22 percent of Americans said that drug abuse had been a cause of trouble in their families. A Pew Foundation poll in 2001 found that 44 percent of Americans were "very concerned" about the possibility of a family member becoming involved with drugs. Another 13 percent were "somewhat concerned." Only 25 percent said they were "not at all concerned."

Q & A

Question: What do parents think influences teen drug use?

Answer: In a Pew Foundation survey in 2002, parents named peer pressure as the most important factor in determining whether or not a teen tries illegal drugs. Other factors of concern to parents included a lack of parental supervision and whether the teen's parents smoke or drank.

Parents are also aware of the influence that they have on teen drug and alcohol use. In the 2001 Pew Foundation survey, 79 percent of Americans said that lack of parental supervision is a major factor affecting a teen's decision to use illegal drugs. Over one-half (52 percent) said that whether the teen's parents smoke or drink also affects the likelihood of teen substance abuse.

While most parents express concern about the possibility of a child becoming involved with drugs, low-income parents (parents in families earning less than $25,000 per year) seem to have greater fears than high-income parents (parents earning more than $75,000 per year). According to a 2002 survey by Public Agenda, 73 percent of low-income parents said they worried "a lot" about protecting their children from drugs and alcohol, compared to 46 percent of high-income parents. However, over one-half (54 percent) of high-income parents named protecting their children from negative societal influences as the biggest challenge they faced in raising their family. Only 42 percent of low-income parents expressed similar views.

Codependence

Despite parental concerns, some teens do take drugs and their use of drugs affects the entire family. How family members react to drug abuse can play a major role in determining the course of abuse. Some family members may become codependent. They may behave in ways that actually support the drug abuse. **Codependence** is a set of compulsive behaviors that develop between a family member and a person within the family who is addicted to drugs. Codependence harms both the person abusing substances and the codependent family member. Codependency may lead to other psychological problems.

DRUG ABUSE AND THE COMMUNITY

Families clearly exert a significant influence on teen drug and alcohol use, but families don't exist in a vacuum. The family is set in a community that includes not only its immediate surroundings but also the larger rural or urban area in which the neighborhood is located. While the city and countryside differ in some respects, both experience the problem of drug and alcohol abuse.

Drugs and community decay

Newspapers and newscasts across the nation reveal the negative effects illegal drug use have on a community. For example, the use of crack (a potent form of cocaine produced by removing cutting agents and other chemicals) struck many cities and towns in the 1980s and 1990s and led to an increase in poverty, crime, and physical decay.

Several studies from the 1980s and 1990s documented the relationship between drug sales in a community and neighborhood decay. A 1990 report, "Drug Marketing, Property Crime, and Neighborhood Viability: Organized Crime Connections," found a relationship between property crimes and drug sales. The study also found that drug sales increased crime and violence in the community and that many people were afraid to use public spaces. Those who could afford to move out did so, leaving behind the poorer residents to face the growing problems.

As the number of abandoned houses grows, property values fall and buildings fall into disrepair. In a 1982 article in *Atlantic Monthly* titled "Breaking Windows," political scientist James Q. Wilson argued that these run-down neighborhoods send the message that they are unsafe places. The climate of fear surrounding such neighborhoods fosters continued crime, violence, and drug use.

According to the 2002 National Crime Victimization Survey, 29 percent of victims of violent crime reported that the offender was using drugs or alcohol at the time of the crime. In 1998 the Bureau of Justice Statistics (BJS) estimated that 61,000 current jail inmates had committed their crimes to obtain money for drugs. The BJS also reported that 8.8 percent of all violent criminals had committed their crimes to get drug money. Violent crime and property crime related to drug use contributes to the decay of neighborhoods and communities.

Urban and suburban drug use
Some people believe that drug use is a problem largely confined to urban areas. To some extent, they are correct. Large cities do experience more problems related to drug abuse. For example, the 1997 National Youth Gang Survey reported that youth gangs were more

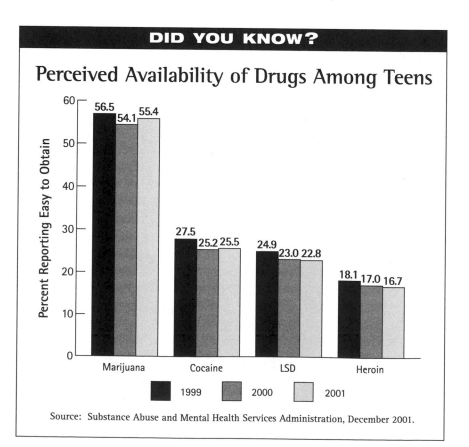

DID YOU KNOW?

Perceived Availability of Drugs Among Teens

Percent Reporting Easy to Obtain

Marijuana: 56.5, 54.1, 55.4
Cocaine: 27.5, 25.2, 25.5
LSD: 24.9, 23.0, 22.8
Heroin: 18.1, 17.0, 16.7

1999   2000   2001

Source: Substance Abuse and Mental Health Services Administration, December 2001.

active in drug sales in larger cities than in small cites or rural areas. Youth gangs were involved in about 49 percent of drug sales in large cities, as compared to 31 percent in small cities and 35 percent in rural areas. These numbers clearly show that suburbs and small towns are not free of drug-related crime.

The survey also showed that youth gangs were involved in 43 percent of drug sales in suburban areas. And a 1995–1996 survey of public high school students taken by the Department of Health and Human Services found that suburban teens were just as likely to drink and use illegal drugs as teens living in urban areas.

Community action

Sociologists and law enforcement professionals have studied ways that communities can work to prevent or decrease local drug use and sales. Studies have shown that enforcing social norms, increasing social interaction, and developing a stronger sense of community can reduce crimes like drug selling. The use of local block watches or neighborhood patrols can reduce drug sales by increasing the seller's risk of getting caught.

For example, people in Seattle organized a watch program in which residents volunteered to ride through the neighborhood, observing and photographing drug sellers and their customers. Although the citizens involved in the program received threats from the drug sellers, they were never actually assaulted. When the volunteers continued to photograph drug deals despite the threats, the sellers left the neighborhood. Other citizen watch programs have had similar successes in reducing drug sales. These efforts show that by working together citizens can help reduce drug sales and drug-related crime in their communities.

Prevention efforts

Communities can also help stop drug abuse before it starts, through programs designed to encourage teens to avoid drugs. Sponsored by schools, churches, and community groups such as the Young Men's Christian Association, these prevention programs aim to reduce or eliminate known risk factors for drug abuse and enhance factors that diminish the potential for drug use. Included in the list of these factors might be:

- A strong positive family environment
- Parental monitoring that is supportive and not overbearing

- Clear rules of conduct that are evenly and consistently enforced
- Parental involvement in their children's lives
- Academic success
- Active membership in quality school and religious groups
- Valuing drug-free beliefs and behaviors

Risk factors for drug use include:

- A chaotic home situation with parents abusing drugs or dealing with mental illness
- Parents with poor parenting skills
- Inappropriately shy or aggressive behavior in school
- Poor academic performance
- Poor **social skills**
- Peers who use drugs
- An acceptance of drug use by family, coworkers, teachers, peers, and others in the community

Fact Or Fiction?

Fear messages stop teens from using drugs.

Fact: Fear messages—actions or communications intended to scare teens away from risky behaviors—have an impact on a teen's behavior. The problem is that after a couple of weeks, the impact of the message wears off. Reinforcement of the message through other means such as classroom discussions, the media, or other activities may extend its impact.

The NIDA suggests that school-based prevention programs include general life skills training and training in resistance skills to strengthen personal attitudes and improve communication skills, peer relationships, self-efficacy, and assertiveness.

Programs designed specifically for teens should include age-appropriate activities including peer discussion groups, group problem solving, and decision making. The institute believes prevention programs should also teach parents or caregivers sound parenting strategies, how to reinforce what their children learn about drugs and their harmful effects, and utilize opportunities for family discussions about drugs and family policies about their use. The institute recommends that prevention programs should continue throughout a child's school years, with practice sessions yearly to reinforce the original goals.

Research on the effectiveness of various prevention programs is very sparse and largely inconclusive. The guidelines above are provided to allow an assessment of various programs and do not imply an endorsement of any specific program. The best program is one that addresses the needs of teens in the local community and that will encourage participation by engaging the concerns and interest of teens and their parents.

TEENS SPEAK

My Friends and I Are Tired of Hearing the Same Old Drug Stories

My name is Julia. The stories we heard at school were all the same. They claimed that someone died from doing this drug or how another drug turned a kid into a vegetable. The stories seemed so bogus.

That all changed the night Pat died. Pat was one of the coolest people at school. He was smart and a great athlete. He was one of those truly rare people who could fit in equally well with the nerds, jocks, and druggies. To say Pat was popular would be an understatement.

Pat didn't believe that drugs were dangerous. One night he had a few beers at a buddy's house and then went on to a party where he took some kind of tablet. He got depressed and then went into a coma and died later that night at the hospital. None of us could figure out what happened. Pat had used the same drug before with no problems and certainly the few beers couldn't have caused such a disaster.

At our next health class, the teacher we all thought was straight-laced and uninformed explained what happened to

Pat that night. The drug Pat took was one made in an underground laboratory. These labs are notorious for having no quality control. As a result, the effects of taking even one tablet can be different from the impact of another tablet of the same drug. Pat took a dose that was much stronger than the drug normally would be. When it reacted with the alcohol in his body, the reaction was strong enough to cause respiratory failure. Without emergency help, Pat slipped into a coma and died. The circumstances had to be right for this to happen, but with underground drugs you never really know exactly what you're getting.

I came away from the story of Pat's death with some new feelings. First, any illegal drug can have unknown consequences, especially when mixed with alcohol. And second, maybe those health teachers aren't so uninformed after all.

See also: Dependence and Addiction; Drugs and Criminal Activity; Risk Factors and Risk Taking

FURTHER READING
Biggers, Jeff. *Chemical Dependency and the Dysfunctional Family.* New York: Rosen Publishing Group, 1998.
Davis, Robert C., Arthur J. Lurigio, and Dennis P. Rosenbaum (ed.). *Drugs and the Community: Involving Community Residents in Combating the Sale of Illegal Drugs.* Springfield, IL: Charles C. Thomas Publishers, Ltd., 1993.
Marlow, Alan. *Young People, Drugs, and Community Safety.* Lyme Regis, UK: Russell House Publishing, Ltd., 1999.
Stimmel, Barry. *The Facts about Drug Use: Coping with Drugs and Alcohol in Your Family, at Work, in Your Community.* Binghamton, NY: The Haworth Press, 1993.

■ GANGS AND DRUGS

Criminal organizations whose members associate for mutual protection and profit from illegal activities. Gangs have been involved in the illicit drug trade for years, but their presence has grown significantly over the past several decades. The reasons for this dramatic increase in gang activity are not completely clear, though many observers point to economic causes. A massive downturn in the economy during the 1980s caused many inner-city blue-collar workers to lose their jobs with little hope for future employment. It is thought that many of these displaced workers found opportunities in gangs.

Crack is a very pure form of cocaine produced by removing cutting agents and other chemicals. The highly addictive drug was sold at a relatively low cost in virtually every city. Crack quickly became the drug of choice because of its rapid effects, low cost, and easy accessibility. The quick rise in use was accompanied by a massive increase in supply by Columbian drug dealers and other producers. As the drug became more popular, gangs that dealt in drugs needed more sales people and tighter controls on their territories. Many gangs became local distributors who controlled millions of dollars in sales.

TRAFFICKING IN DRUGS

According to the Office of Juvenile Justice and Delinquency Prevention (OJJDP), in 1997 approximately 33 percent of the teen gangs in the United States were involved in drug trafficking. About 57 percent of these gangs were in the larger cities. The National Youth Gang Survey defines trafficking as "the purchase or transfer of large quantities of drugs which are divided into smaller quantities to be sold on the street." Street sales refer to the distribution of small quantities of drugs to individual users.

The OJJDP also reported that 42 percent of teen gangs were involved in the street sale of drugs. Statistics from across the country suggest that roughly 33 percent of crack cocaine sales, 32 percent of marijuana sales, 16 percent of powder cocaine sales, 12 percent of methamphetamine sales, and 9 percent of heroin sales were through gangs. Gangs generated incredible profits through the sale of drugs and used those profits to entice teens to become gang members.

Not only have teen gangs played a huge role in the sale of drugs, but research also suggests that their role in trafficking may be substantial as well. Trafficking through the movement of gangs to new communities is a major concern of law enforcement. According to the National Youth Gang Survey, 18 percent of all youth gang members had moved to their current residence from another area. Migration beyond the territory or region of the gang can establish new markets and expand sales, thus increasing drug purchases and profits. Many gangs have migrated into small cities and rural towns.

Percentage of Youth Gangs Involved in Street Drug Sales, by Region

Region	Total Gangs	Drug Gangs	
		Number	Percent
Midwest	2,749	1,253	46%
Northeast	768	463	60
South	4,242	1,753	41
West	5,484	999	18
Overall	13,243	4,468	34

Source: National Youth Gang Survey, Office of Juvenile Justice and Delinquency Prevention, 1998.

The trade in illegal drugs is much like legitimate businesses in that both want to increase market share and profits, protect their sales territory, and keep employees motivated. The obvious difference is that gangs sell an illegal product and use fear, violence, and murder to accomplish their goals.

Fact Or Fiction?

Youth gangs in larger cities are more involved in drug sales than gangs in smaller towns.

Fact: According to the 1997 National Youth Gang Survey, almost one-half (49 percent) of the youth gangs in cities with more than 100,000 people were involved in drug sales. Only 29 percent of youth gangs were involved in drug sales in towns with fewer than 10,000 residents.

DRUG ABUSE AMONG GANG MEMBERS

Recent studies have provided insights into the inner workings of gangs, including drug use by gang members. It seems to vary widely from gang to gang. In a 1998 paper titled "Addressing Community Gang Problems: A Practical Guide," the Department of Justice reported that different gangs have different attitudes toward drug use by members. Some gangs prohibit drug use by members. In other cases, it is not specifically forbidden but is frowned on. For example, Dr. Pamela LaBorde of the University of Washington Harborview Medical Center reported that while many Vietnamese gangs sell heroin, few gang members use drugs. They consider heroin users weak. Each gang seems to have unwritten guidelines related to drug use.

GANG-RELATED HOMICIDE

Violence and drugs have been intricately linked, and the violence often results in homicide. A 1997 survey by the OJJDP estimated that youth gang members were involved in some 3,340 homicides. The vast majority of those murders took place in large cities. Teen gang involvement in other types of criminal activity remained high in 1997: Gangs were involved in 28 percent of all aggravated assaults and larceny/theft crimes, 27 percent of motor vehicle thefts, 26 percent of burglaries, and 13 percent of all robberies.

The number of gang homicides is closely tied to territorial disputes and the ever-present threat of losing ground to a rival gang, which would mean a drop in drug sales and profits. Because virtually every gang wants to generate more profits, each tries to not only protect its own territory but also to expand into the territories of rival gangs. Law enforcement may inadvertently increase the tension. For example, if the police set out to drive drug dealers from First Street, they may force the dealers to move to Second Street. However, if Second Street is in another gang's territory, a drug war is likely to begin.

Another important issue regarding homicide and gangs is the availability of handguns. In its 2001 *Juvenile Justice Bulletin* the OJJDP reported that gang members are twice as likely as other teens to carry a weapon. Whether to defend themselves from rivals, ensure a smooth drug transaction, or simply defend their honor against someone who disrespected them, gang members use guns frequently.

See also: Drugs and Criminal Activity; Homicide

■ HOMICIDE

Homicide, or murder, is the intentional taking of another person's life. Homicide is the second-leading cause of death among teens between the ages of 15 and 19. According to the Office of Juvenile Justice and

Delinquency Prevention (OJJDP), homicide claimed the lives of more than 1,200 teens in the United States in 1999. Although that number represents a decline from previous years, the rate of teen homicide in the United States is still significantly higher than in any other Western nation.

CRIMES COMMITTED UNDER THE INFLUENCE
According to "Violence and Drug Abuse," a 1995 publication by the National Institute on Drug Abuse (NIDA), approximately 50 percent of violent crimes can be attributed to alcohol abuse. Some 30 percent of these violent crimes are homicides. Alcohol increases aggressiveness and decreases inhibitions, an explosive combination that can lead to violence. **Cocaine** and **methamphetamines** also have the reputation of generating feelings of aggression and hostility. Statistics from the Federal Bureau of Investigation's Uniform Crime Reports show that less than 5 percent of all homicides are related to drugs other than alcohol.

A major issue in teen homicide is the accessibility of firearms. In the Federal Interagency Forum on Child and Family Statistics' 1999 publication "America's Children: Key National Indicators of Well-Being," firearms were identified as the instrument of death in over 80 percent of teen homicides in 1999. "The Future of Children," a publication of the Woodrow Wilson School of Public Affairs at Princeton University, reports that roughly one in four teen deaths results from firearm injuries, while only one in 760 teen deaths results from non-firearm injuries. With access to firearms, a teen's momentary anger or carelessness can end in tragedy. Under the influence of alcohol or illicit drugs, the chances of this happening increase.

Many of the homicides committed by teens are against other teens. According to the OJJDP, in 1997 juveniles killed 25 percent of all homicide victims under the age of 18, and almost all of those young killers were teens. Firearms were involved in 74 percent of those murders, and in 68 percent of the cases, the victims knew their killers.

Fact Or Fiction?

Homicide rates are about the same for most ethnic groups.

Fact: Homicide affects certain populations at a much higher rate than other groups. Statistics from 2000 show that black male teens have a much higher homicide rate (57.9 deaths per 100,000 population) than Hispanic males (29 per 100,000), Native Americans (18 per 100,000) or white males (3.4 per 100,000). Black females also have higher homicide rates than females of other races. The rate among black females was 8.6 per 100,000 compared to 3.1 for Hispanic females and 1.9 for white females.

No single fact explains the higher rates of homicide among black teens, especially black males. The data does, however, show an association between income and teen homicide. According to the 2000 U.S. Census, African Americans had the lowest yearly median income ($29,470) among any ethnic group. Black income was significantly below the figure for white households ($46,305), and it also trails both Hispanics ($33,500) and Native Americans ($32,000).

CRIMES COMMITTED IN TRAFFICKING

Drug trafficking—the distribution and sale of drugs—has become a principal effort of gangs in the United States. So it should come as no surprise that violence, specifically homicide, is a part of gang membership. Gang violence has been associated with many teen murders. According to "Homicides of Children and Youth," an article published by the OJJDP, in 1997 nearly 30 percent of teen homicides were attributed to gang violence.

During the 1980s, the sharp rise in illegal drug use—particularly the introduction of crack, a potent form of cocaine produced by removing cutting agents and other chemicals—led drug traffickers to hire more dealers. Gang leaders began to recruit teens, because they worked more cheaply than adults and because many of the adults who once sold drugs were in prison. Many teens eagerly signed on, despite the dangers involved. The growth in firearm use among teenage gang members has led to an increase in guns and other weapons in the community at large. As a result, the rise in homicide among gang members was soon matched by a similar rise among teens in general.

As the epidemic of crack use subsided in the early-to-mid-1990s, the rate of teen homicide also declined, as has the number of teens involved in drug trafficking. A rise in teen employment, especially among minority youth, encouraged many teens to turn away from drug trafficking. As a result, teen homicide has declined significantly since the mid-1990s.

Despite the recent declines in gang violence, gang activity still claims many teenage victims. The OJJDP estimated that in 1997 youth gang members were involved in some 3,340 homicides. Gangs were involved in 26 percent of teen homicides and drugs were involved in 6 percent. The OJJDP reports that the territories most frequently fought for are in large cities. This is probably due to the greater potential market for drug sales in larger cities. Territorial disputes and the threat of losing turf to rival gangs can represent a drop in drug sales. And in certain respects drug trafficking is not much different than any other enterprise that needs to expand and generate increased profits. Like legitimate businesses, drug traffickers are concerned about protecting their existing markets.

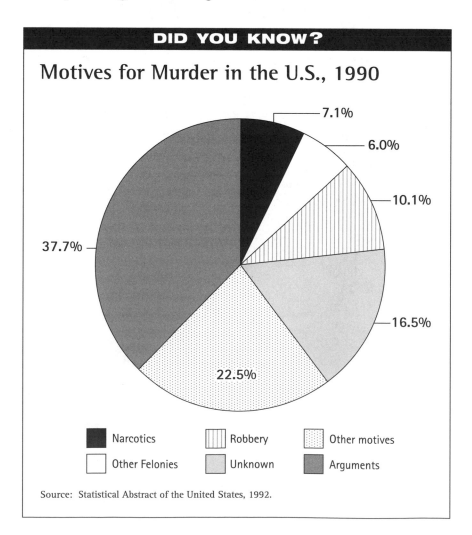

DID YOU KNOW?

Motives for Murder in the U.S., 1990

7.1%

6.0%

10.1%

37.7%

16.5%

22.5%

■ Narcotics   ▥ Robbery   ▦ Other motives

□ Other Felonies   ▨ Unknown   ▩ Arguments

Source: Statistical Abstract of the United States, 1992.

Loss of turf to a rival gang can also lead a tarnished reputation, another significant source of gang violence. The losing gang often decides to retaliate with violence against their rivals. This may well include killing a rival gang member, an act that can fuel a desire for revenge and lead to a continued cycle of homicide. This cycle of provocation, retaliation, and revenge fuels most gang violence.

Gang members carry weapons for a variety of reasons, from defending themselves from a rival gang, to assuring a smooth drug transaction, to defending their reputation against anyone who disrespects them. Firearms are the weapon of choice in gang-related violence. In fact, from the mid-1980s to the mid-1990s—a period that saw a dramatic increase in teen homicide—virtually the entire increase was due to the rise in firearm violence. Gangs involved in drug trafficking committed much of that violence.

RISKS TO USERS

Drug users are more likely than nonusers to be victims of homicide, especially if they are associated with a gang. Gang involvement in drug trafficking is big business. However, **street sale** of drugs, not trafficking, is the primary business of most gangs. The OJJDP reported that 42 percent of teen gangs are involved in the street sale of drugs. Statistics from across the country suggest that roughly 33 percent of crack cocaine sales, 32 percent of **marijuana** sales, 16 percent of powder cocaine sales, 12 percent of **methamphetamine** sales, and 9 percent of **heroin** sales are through gangs.

RATES

According to the Child Trend Data Bank, between 1970 and 1993 the homicide rate for teens ages 15–19 more than doubled, from 7.7 to 20.5 per 100,000. Between 1993 and 2000, the rate declined dramatically. In 1993, just over 20 of every 100,000 teens in the United States was a victim of homicide. In 2000, only 9.6 of every 100,000 teens died as a result of homicide. These most recent numbers may be related to a reduction in firearm use. Recent statistics show that firearm-related deaths have similarly declined, falling to 13.1 per 100,000 in 2000 from a high of 28 per 100,000 in 1995.

Combined with the reduction in firearm violence is a corresponding drop in the use of alcohol and illicit drugs among teens. A 2003 survey by NIDA noted a decline in the percentage of teens who had ever used alcohol or illicit drugs since 1997. Both of these trends—

declining firearm violence and a drop in drug use—offer hope for a continued reduction in teen homicide.

See also: Drugs and Criminal Activity; Drugs and Drinking; Gangs and Drugs

■ ILLEGAL DRUGS, COMMON

Widely used drugs whose manufacture, sale, and use are prohibited by law. Also called illicit drugs, these are the substances that most teens generally refer to as "drugs." The illegal drugs most commonly used by teens represent a range of substances with widely varying physical and behavioral effects. Some depress the central nervous system, causing drowsiness, impaired judgment, and lack of coordination. Others stimulate the user, producing a heightened state of alertness, anxiety, and nervousness. The effects of some of these drugs last only a few minutes, while others linger for several hours. The one thing they share is that all cause changes in the body's chemistry—changes that alter the user's perceptions.

MARIJUANA

Marijuana—commonly referred to as "grass," "weed," or "pot"—is a drug derived from the dried flowers and leaves of the plant *Cannabis sativa*. Marijuana is usually rolled into cigarettes (joints) and smoked. Marijuana may also be smoked in a pipe ordinarily used for tobacco or in a water pipe ("bong").

Typically, the effects of marijuana take hold within 10 to 30 minutes and last approximately three hours. Although effects differ, marijuana generally affects memory and learning, distorts perception, and results in difficulty in thinking and problem solving, a loss of coordination, and an increased heart rate. Marijuana can also alter mood and distort the way the user experiences sight, sound, and his or her other senses.

Marijuana has been used for thousands of years, but it did not gain widespread popularity in the United States until the 1960s. However, today's marijuana is much more potent than the marijuana of the 1960s. By some estimates it is two to five times as strong. These more potent strains of marijuana are produced by selective breeding of certain plants to increase the concentration of the drug's active ingredient, delta-9 tetrahyrocannibinol, or THC.

Marijuana use among teens increased throughout the 1960s and 1970s, reaching a peak in the mid-1970s. After a decline in the 1980s, the number of teens using marijuana climbed again during the 1990s, reaching a peak in 1998 and 1999. Since that time, both the number of teens who have ever smoked marijuana and those who smoke it regularly have been on the decline.

Many teens believe that marijuana is a relatively safe drug with few harmful side effects. However, a number of studies show that marijuana use can be dangerous. One study by the National Institute on Drug Abuse (NIDA) showed that marijuana impaired the ability to operate a car safely. The study indicated that marijuana was implicated in almost half of all accidents involving drivers under the age of 30. In addition, long-term marijuana smokers often experienced chronic (long-term) conditions similar to those suffered by cigarette smokers, including lung damage and suppression of the immune system.

TEENS SPEAK

Marijuana Is Not As It Seems

I'm Manny and I often hear teens saying that marijuana should be legalized because they know a lot of teens who smoke and nothing bad has happened to them. I also hear them say that even if the cops get you, they consider the crime small because they want the big kingpins who are trafficking in heavy drugs.

But I tell them they're stupid if they use grass. I should know; my brother Ben used to use it all the time. He started when he was about 13, and I could tell right away that it was affecting his brain. Before he started smoking weed he was a good student, but afterwards he had trouble remembering things. He was also a good athlete at one time; he played on the football, basketball, and baseball teams in middle school. After Ben began to smoke weed, he lost his focus and interest and he couldn't make any of the teams in high school.

Ben started hanging out and cruising around with a bunch of other guys who smoked. One day Ben was driving home stoned and he ran a red light. The crash killed him instantly and hurt the driver of the other car. Ben never would have had that crash if he hadn't been high; he probably would have been practicing sports instead of driving around stoned and wasting time. After Ben's death, I never pass up an opportunity to tell other kids that marijuana is dangerous, so don't let some uninformed big mouth tell you that nothing bad happens when you do grass. They are wrong, dead wrong.

COCAINE

Cocaine is a white powder produced by chemically treating the leaves of the coca plant. Coca leaves contain a natural stimulant that is released when the leaves are chewed. South American Indians have long used raw coca as a source of quick energy. Raw coca undergoes several chemical processes before the extract of the leaves are transformed into the white powder called cocaine. Cocaine can be snorted, smoked, or injected.

Cocaine has profound and contradictory effects. It stimulates the central nervous system, making the user more alert, active, and nervous. However, it also has anesthetic or pain-killing qualities. Its effects can include mood elevation, a decrease in fatigue, an increase in alertness, and greater self-confidence. However, these effects are temporary. Increased amounts of the substance produce irritability, apprehensiveness, paranoia, and violent behaviors. Physical effects of cocaine use include increased heart rate, elevated blood pressure, loss of appetite, convulsions, muscle twitching, irregular heartbeat, and, possibly, death.

Snorting cocaine can damage the lining of the nose, cause sinus infection, and impact the sense of smell. Smoking or "freebasing" cocaine can cause liver and lung damage. Cocaine can also burn uncontrollably when exposed to fire, and accidents involving freebasing have resulted in serious burns. Injecting cocaine carries the negative consequences of injecting any drug, the most serious being HIV infection (a virus that attacks the body's immune system and causes AIDS) and hepatitis (infectious disease that can cause serious liver damage). In addition, cocaine is often mixed, or "cut" with other chemicals, including other stimulants, that can have adverse effects of their own.

Q & A

Question: What is "freebasing"?

Answer: Freebase is the most powerful form of cocaine. It is produced by mixing powdered cocaine with volatile chemicals like ether. This process removes the hydrochloride salts used to make powder cocaine from raw coca leaves. It also removes "cutting agents"—substances such as amphetamines that are often mixed into powder cocaine before it is sold. The result is a pure form of cocaine that is usually smoked through a water pipe or heated on a piece of foil with a lighter. Users inhale the resulting smoke. The freebase rush is quick, intense, and over quickly, which makes it highly addictive and more powerful than powder cocaine or crack.

A particularly potent form of cocaine called **crack** is produced by removing cutting agents and other chemicals. This process creates a dense mass, or "rock," of cocaine that is roughly 90 percent pure. When smoked, crack provides an intense high that lasts about 20 minutes and is followed immediately by depression, edginess, and a craving for more of the drug. The intense high in the limited time period keeps crack users coming back. Although crack is relatively inexpensive, the need to continually achieve the high has resulted in drug habits costing thousands of dollars per day.

Statistics complied by NIDA show that the use of both cocaine and crack cocaine among teens increased steadily from 1991 to 2001. However, the trend seems to be reversing. Since 2002 the use of both powder and crack cocaine among teens has declined steadily.

HEROIN

Heroin is a drug produced from morphine, a chemical that occurs naturally in the seeds of the Asian poppy plant. It is part of a family of drugs called **opiates**, which generally cause drowsiness, relieve pain, and produce **euphoria** (an intense sense of well-being). Until recently, almost all users injected heroin, but the increased potency of today's heroin enables users to snort or smoke it. Nevertheless, most users continue to inject the drug, a process referred to as "mainlining."

The short-term effects of heroin abuse appear quickly and fade in a few hours. Users typically feel a surge of euphoria, accompanied by a warm flush of the skin, dry mouth, and heaviness in the arms and legs. This is followed by an alternately wakeful and drowsy state caused by a depression of the central nervous system that clouds mental functioning.

Long-term effects may include collapsed veins, infection of the heart, and liver disease. By depressing breathing, heroin use can also lead to pneumonia and other problems with the pulmonary system (the system that delivers oxygen to the body). Heroin may also contain additives that can clog blood vessels leading to the lungs, liver, kidneys, or brain. The clotting can kill cells and cause infections in vital organs. Intravenous heroin use, as with cocaine, has also been shown to increase the risk of HIV infection, hepatitis B, and hepatitis C.

Heroin use increased dramatically during the 1990s. In 1997, NIDA reported that there were 81,000 new heroin users, and between 1990 and 1995 the number of heroin-related emergency room visits doubled. The increased use of heroin came at a time when supplies increased and prices fell. Nevertheless, heroin remains extremely addictive and treatment efforts have had limited success.

CLUB AND DESIGNER DRUGS

The terms *club drugs* and *designer drugs* refer to a wide range of synthetic substances from a variety of drug categories. The club drug roster includes ecstasy (MDMA), GHB (gammahydroxybutyrate), roofies (Rohypnol), and Special K (ketamine). Club and designer drugs typically are produced in underground laboratories. These labs vary greatly in the quality of the drugs they produce and in the potency of a single dose. No one knows exactly what chemicals were used and in what quantities.

Ecstasy and Special K are examples of club drugs that have stimulant effects. The effects of ecstasy are similar to those of **amphetamines**: increased alertness and energy sometimes accompanied by euphoria and **hallucinations** (false or distorted perceptions). Ecstasy has gained popularity because of its reputation for heightening sexual pleasure and reducing the user's sensitivity to pain. However, users face many of the same risks as users of other stimulants, such as increased heart rate and blood pressure, muscle tension, nausea, blurred vision, faintness, and chills or sweating. More seriously, these drugs can cause a sharp increase in body temperature (hyperthermia) leading to failure of the liver, kidney, and cardiovascular system. Psychological effects can include confusion, depression, sleep problems, and severe anxiety.

The effects of Special K are similar to those of ecstasy but are not as severe, a factor that has added to its popularity.

By contrast, GHB and Rohypnol act as **depressants**, causing drowsiness, confusion, and impaired judgment and motor coordination. Rohypnol—commonly known as the **date rape drug**—causes a **sedative** effect within 20 to 30 minutes. It dissolves quickly in alcohol and, when secretly slipped into someone's drink, can quickly render a person unconscious, making him or her helpless against sexual assault. The victim may also have great difficulty remembering what happened under the influence of the drug. GHB is also a sedative that has also been used as a date rape drug. Mixing GHB with other drugs such as alcohol can result in nausea and difficulty breathing. GHB may also produce **withdrawal** effects, including insomnia, anxiety, and tremors.

Teen use of club and designer drugs increased dramatically during the 1990s, reaching a peak around 2000. The numbers began to decline thereafter, but the percentage of teens using ecstasy in 2003 was still three times as high as it was in 1996.

BARBITURATES

Barbiturates, such as mephobarbital (Mebaral) and pentobarbital sodium (Nembutal), are central nervous system depressants used to treat anxiety, tension, and sleep disorders. They typically are taken in pill form. When consumed in small doses, they result in a lack of responsiveness and muscular coordination. In higher doses they can cause slurred speech, decreased rate of breathing, slowed heart rate, unconsciousness, and death. If taken with alcohol even in small doses, the combination can cause respiratory functions to slow down to such an extent that death can occur. Barbiturates are extremely addictive and typically require medical intervention to overcome.

AMYL NITRATE

Amyl nitrate is a drug that reduces blood pressure and causes the blood vessels to expand rapidly, which is why it is used to reduce chest pain in heart patients. It is believed to enhance sexual sensations and orgasm by increasing blood flow to the genitals. Physical effects include headache, flushing of the face, decreased blood pressure, increased pulse, dizziness, and the relaxation of certain muscles—especially the blood vessel walls and the anal sphincter (a circular muscle that opens and closes the anus). Teen use is less than

1 percent, according to the University of Michigan's 1999 study "Monitoring the Future."

AMPHETAMINES

Amphetamines such as benzoamphetamine (Benzedrine) and dextroamphetamine (Dexedrine) are synthetically produced stimulants that have the opposite effect of barbiturates. Amphetamines go by a wide array of names, including bennies, dexies, and speed. Amphetamines in small doses improve alertness, reduce fatigue, and elevate mood. In larger quantities over extended periods of time they can cause a laundry list of problems, including hallucinations and paranoia. They are, however, a category of illegal drugs that do have medical uses. For example, methylphenidate (Ritalin) is used to treat ADHD (attention deficit hyperactive disorder) and fenfluramine hydrochloride (Pondimin) is used to treat obesity.

Methamphetamines—also known as ice, meth, and crank—are a family of nervous system stimulants related to amphetamines that produce similar but much more intense effects. Methamphetamine comes in a powder form that can be snorted, smoked or taken orally or by intravenous injection. Because the drug is produced in illegal laboratories, it may include other dangerous chemicals used in processing.

The effects of taking even small amounts of methamphetamine include increased wakefulness and physical activity, decreased appetite, rapid breathing, hyperthermia, and euphoria. Immediately after smoking or injection, the user experiences an intensely pleasurable sensation, or "rush," that lasts just a few minutes. Oral or nasal use produces euphoria but not the intense rush caused by injection or snorting. Other effects include irritability, insomnia, confusion, tremors, convulsions, anxiety, paranoia, and aggressiveness. Hyperthermia and convulsions can result in death. Long-term use can cause increased heart rate and blood pressure and irreversible damage to blood vessels in the brain, leading to stroke. Respiratory problems, irregular heartbeat, and extreme anorexia can also occur, and continued use can result in cardiovascular collapse and death.

Methamphetamines have gained popularity because of their physical effects and lengthy high, which can last from four to 14 hours. These drugs are often used by people who need to stay alert for many hours, such as long-distance truck drivers, people who work all-night shifts, and students cramming for examinations. Overall use among teens has risen gradually since the mid-1990s.

HALLUCINOGENS

Hallucinogens are drugs that cause the user to experience distorted sights, sounds, and other sensations. These distorted sensations are called hallucinations. Some hallucinogens, such as lysergic acid diethalymide (**LSD**) are synthetic while others, such as peyote and mescaline, are derived from natural plant sources. Most hallucinogens are taken orally. For example, LSD (also called acid) comes in several forms but is primarily sold as small squares of blotter paper saturated with the drug, which are chewed or swallowed.

Hallucinogens distort the user's sense of reality, causing him or her to hear, feel, and see things that aren't there. Flashbacks—the reexperiencing of drug effects from previous uses—have been known to occur months or years after using hallucinogens. Other effects associated with hallucinogen use include depression, muscular weakness, anxiety or paranoia, trembling, nausea, and dizziness. The impact of hallucinogens can vary dramatically from one episode to another. Because of the effects these drugs have on heart rate and blood pressure, the results of continued use can be coma, lung, and/or heart failure. Users often suffer from feelings of confusion, suspicion, and disorientation, which may cause speech problems, weird body movements, and aggressive or violent behavior.

Unlike marijuana, which is more potent today than it was in the 1970s, the strength of the average dose of LSD has decreased since that time. Nevertheless, there is still a high potential for adverse effects, even with reduced dosages. Teen use of LSD increased during the mid-1990s but has been in steady decline since about 1997.

PCP

Phencyclidine, or **PCP**, is a depressant that affects the central nervous system. It was originally used as an anesthetic to eliminate pain during medical procedures while the patient remained conscious. Its medical use was discontinued in 1965 because patients often became agitated, delusional, and irrational while recovering from its effects. Today the drug is mostly produced in illegal laboratories. Also known as angel dust, PCP is a white powder that can be taken orally or snorted, and is frequently sprinkled onto marijuana joints.

At low to moderate doses, the physical effects of PCP include a slight increase in breathing rate and a dramatic rise in blood pressure and pulse rate. Shallow breathing, flushing of the skin, and heavy sweating can also occur, accompanied by numbness in the arms and

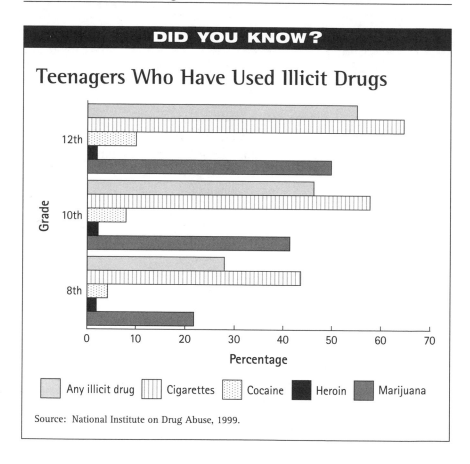

DID YOU KNOW?

Teenagers Who Have Used Illicit Drugs

Legend: Any illicit drug, Cigarettes, Cocaine, Heroin, Marijuana

Source: National Institute on Drug Abuse, 1999.

legs and loss of muscular coordination. Taking PCP with other central nervous system depressants such as alcohol or barbiturates can lead to coma or accidental overdose. At high doses, blood pressure, pulse rate, and respiration drop. Nausea, vomiting, blurred vision, drooling, loss of balance, and dizziness can also occur. High doses of PCP can also cause seizures, coma, and death (usually from accidental injury or suicide rather than as a direct effect of the drug).

Extreme psychological effects of PCP use resemble symptoms of **schizophrenia**, including **delusions**, hallucinations, paranoia, disordered thinking, a sensation of distance from the environment, inability to move, and garbled speech. Long-term use can lead to memory loss, difficulties with speech and thinking, depression, and weight loss. These symptoms can last up to a year after stopping PCP use. Use of PCP among teens is not widespread; in 2002 only about 1 percent of teenagers reported using the drug.

NO SAFE DRUGS

Although illegal drug use among teens has decreased across most categories of drugs, the wide variety and ready availability of such substances poses a serious health threat to teens. All of the drugs discussed in this article have adverse mental and physical effects, and prolonged use of many of these drugs can have serious negative consequences, including death. No drug is "safe," regardless of what your friends may tell you. The short- and long-term risks of drug use are great, and the best strategy for dealing with such drugs is to avoid them altogether.

See also: Crack Cocaine; Drug Abuse, Causes of; Drugs and Disease; Inhalants; Injection Drugs; Sexual Behavior and Drug Abuse

FURTHER READING

Clark, Michael. *Common Illegal Drugs and Their Effects: Cannabis, Ecstasy, Amphetamines, and LSD.* London: The Stationery Office Books, 1996.

Gahlinger, Paul M. *Illegal Drugs: A Complete Guide to Their History, Chemistry, Use, and Abuse.* Las Vegas: Sagebrush Press. 2001.

Robson, Philip. *Forbidden Drugs.* Oxford: Oxford University Press. 1999.

Rudgley, Richard. *The Encyclopedia of Psychoactive Substances.* New York: St. Martin's Press, 1998.

■ INHALANTS

Substances that give off fumes which, when inhaled (taken into the body by breathing), can produce a drug high. The inhalants used today are inexpensive and readily available in most homes, factors that increase their potential for abuse (the nonmedical use of a substance in order to affect one's mental processes, satisfy a dependence, or attempt suicide). They include products such as paint, nail polishes, lighter fluids, refrigerants, glues, aerosols, cleaning solutions, fuels, lighter fluids, PVC (plastic pipe) cement, hair spray, and correction (typing) fluid.

Q & A

Question: If inhalants can be purchased in any store, how can they be harmful?

Answer: Some teens wrongly believe that because inhalants are legal, they are not harmful. Nothing could be further from the truth. If used as intended, these products are safe. When they are inhaled, they can be extremely toxic.

TYPES OF INHALANTS

The National Institute on Drug Abuse (NIDA) classifies inhalants into four basic types, or categories.

- Volatile solvents are liquids that turn into gases at room temperature. They include paint thinners and removers, dry-cleaning fluids, degreasers, gasoline, glues, correction fluids, and felt-tip marker fluids.

- Aerosols are sprays containing propellants and solvents. They include spray paint, spray deodorant, hair spray, vegetable oil sprays for cooking, and fabric protector sprays.

- Gases include medical anesthetics and commercial or household gases. Examples of medical anesthetic gases are ether, chloroform, and nitrous oxide, also called "laughing gas." Nitrous oxide, the most abused of the gases, is also found in whipped cream dispensers. Household or commercial products containing inhalant gases include butane lighters, propane tanks, whipped cream dispensers, and refrigerants.

- Nitrites are a special class of inhalants. Most inhalants affect the central nervous system, but nitrites relax the muscles and dilate blood vessels to increase blood flow. While other inhalants are used to alter mood, nitrites are used primarily to enhance sexual pleasure. Nitrites include cyclohexyl nitrite, which is found in some room deodorizers. Because it increases blood flow to the heart, isoamyl (amyl) nitrite is prescribed for patients with chest pain. Doses of amyl nitrite used for recreation are called "poppers" or "snappers" on the street. Isobutyl (butyl) nitrite is a substance similar to amyl nitrite that is often packaged and sold in small bottles also referred to as "poppers."

EFFECTS OF INHALANTS

Inhalants contain gases that when inhaled or "huffed" produce **euphoria**, dizziness, confusion, and drowsiness. The effect of using inhalants is felt quickly because the user breathes the fumes directly into the lungs. This causes the chemicals in the fumes to reach the bloodstream in seconds, where they are quickly transported to the brain. The euphoric effects from the substance typically last 15 minutes or less. Inhalants irritate the mucous membranes of the eyes, mouth, nose, throat, and lungs, as well as presenting a few unusual concerns for users. These include suffocation from huffing on a plastic bag and the possibility of explosion if the volatile fumes are exposed to a fire or open flame.

Inhalants are dangerous. Abuse of inhalants over a period of time can cause a number of serious health effects. The short-term effects include amnesia, an inability to concentrate, confusion, and impaired judgment. **Hallucinations** are another typical effect of inhalants. Inhalants can also cause long-term health problems such as brain damage, irregular heartbeat, anemia, liver damage, kidney failure, coma, and death. Combining inhalants with alcohol can cause dangerous interactions between the drugs and lead to serious health risks, including severe liver damage and even death.

Inhalants do not produce **tolerance, withdrawal,** or symptoms characteristic of **physical dependence,** and the possibility of **psychological dependence** is limited. A primary concern in the use of inhalants is the inability to control the dose. Because every person's lung capacity is different, it is impossible to control the amount of substance inhaled. If too much of a volatile aerosol is huffed, unconsciousness can occur. If breathing is restricted for any reason while in this unconscious state, death can occur within minutes.

Fact Or Fiction?

There are always specific signs of inhalant use by teens.

Fact: Although use of an inhalant is usually apparent, sometimes it is difficult to tell. If someone you know is exhibiting one or more of the following warning signs, they may be using inhalants:

- Slurred speech
- Drunk, dizzy, or dazed appearance
- Unusual breath odor
- Chemical smell on clothing
- Paint stains on body or face

- Red eyes
- Runny nose

Inhalant use can be dangerous, so if you suspect a friend is doing it, talk with them and seek appropriate help.

The Centers for Disease Control and Prevention reports that in 2001 almost 15 percent of students nationwide had sniffed glue, breathed the contents of aerosol spray cans, or inhaled paints or sprays to get high during their lifetime. However, according to a survey by NIDA, inhalant use by teens in 2003 was at its lowest level since 1991, the first year inhalant use was studied among eighth and 10th graders. The report also stated that rates for 12th graders were the lowest in 20 years. The report did raise concerns about perceived risk (how much risk individuals feel they are taking when they use a drug). Low perceived risk means that users are less concerned about the effects of abuse, an indicator of increased use in the future. Disappointingly, the perceived risk from trying inhalants was low among eighth and 10th graders, indicating the possibility of greater use in years to come.

See also: Dependence and Addiction; Drugs and Drinking; Overdose and Drugs

■ INJECTION DRUGS

Drugs that are taken by injection into either the veins or muscles of the user. Among the most common **intravenous drugs**—drugs administered by injection into a vein—are **heroin** (an illicit drug, derived from the poppy plant, that causes drowsiness, relieves pain, and produces euphoria), **cocaine** (an illicit drug, derived from the coca plant, that increases energy and alertness), and **amphetamines** (synthetically produced stimulants that improve alertness, reduce fatigue, and elevate mood). Until recently, all injection drugs were classified as intravenous drugs. However, that changed with the growing abuse of muscle-building drugs called **anabolic steroids**, which are injected into muscles. The term *injection drug* includes both to cover intravenous and intramuscular drugs.

Intravenous drug use in the past was limited almost exclusively to heroin. Today, heroin is one of several illegal drugs that can be administered by injection. Virtually any drug can be injected if it is dissolved in a liquid solution, but heroin, cocaine, and amphetamines make up the three primary injection drugs.

An intravenous injection introduces drugs instantly into the bloodstream, allowing the drug to reach the brain very quickly. As a result, injections produce effects within minutes. While intravenous use of heroin and other drugs has been of concern for many years, the use of such drugs soared to national attention when their use was found to be directly associated with HIV infection and AIDS. HIV is the virus that causes AIDS (acquired immune deficiency syndrome), a medical condition in which the body's immune system is so weakened that even mild infections can cause death.

Drug users who are infected with HIV can spread the virus by sharing needles with other users. The HIV virus that causes AIDS attacks the immune system and depletes it to such an extent that infections the body typically fights off—like colds or the flu—become life threatening. For persons with AIDS, common infections can be deadly. There is no known cure for HIV or AIDS.

TEENS SPEAK

It's Really Hard to Lose a Friend

It's even harder to lose a friend twice. My name is Carolyn, and I lost my friend Steve twice. The first time I lost him to heroin; the second time I lost him to HIV.

Steve was really a cool guy. He was funny and smart and he kept telling everyone how he was going to be a comedian or an actor. He was always doing really wild things like dyeing his hair green for St. Patrick's Day and wallpapering his locker at school. There wasn't a lot Steve wouldn't at least consider doing for kicks, and that's how he started getting into trouble with drugs.

One day I saw some marks on Steve's arm, and I asked him what they were. When he told me he had tried shooting heroin, I freaked out. I knew how dangerous heroin was, and

I was worried that he'd get addicted. I begged him to stop, but he said I worried too much. But after a while, I could tell I was right. Steve stopped being the fun guy I knew and started spending all of his time wasted. He looked terrible; every time I saw him it was like I was looking at a ghost.

I really began to worry when a couple of months went by and I hadn't seen Steve at all. None of his old friends knew where he was, and I was too afraid to talk to the stoners he used to hang out with. When I called his house, his sister told me he was in the hospital. The doctors said he had HIV and that he most likely got it from sharing an infected needle. His sister said he was sick all the time and he was avoiding all of his old friends. It's been almost six months now since I last saw Steve, and I don't know if he's even still alive. In a way I suppose the Steve I knew died when he started using drugs.

HIV infection is not the only health risk associated with sharing needles. Other blood-borne diseases that can be transmitted by sharing injection drugs include **hepatitis** B and C. Hepatitis attacks the liver, causing a variety of symptoms, including fever, headache, nausea, loss of appetite, skin rashes, and the yellowing of eyes and skin referred to as jaundice. Over time, hepatitis can cause serious persistent liver infections and chronic (long-term) liver disease, which may result in liver cancer and death.

The risk of AIDS or hepatitis is not a side effect of heroin or other injection drugs. Instead it is the result of sharing infected needles. Whenever someone injects a substance into his or her body, blood is always deposited on, and possibly in, the needle. Unless the needles are cleaned thoroughly with bleach, that blood will be injected into the next person who uses the needle. The use of new needles, or the cleaning of used ones, could reduce HIV transmission and hepatitis substantially. However, injection drug users typically share drugs and needles with a close-knit group of people and are often reluctant to ask other users to clean their needles.

In the United States, the role that injection drug use plays in transmitting both HIV and hepatitis is substantial. According to the May 18, 2001 issue of *Morbidity and Mortality Weekly Report* from the Centers for Disease Control and Prevention, roughly 33 percent of AIDS cases and 50 percent of hepatitis C cases are attributable to injection drug use. The report also stated that some 1 million people

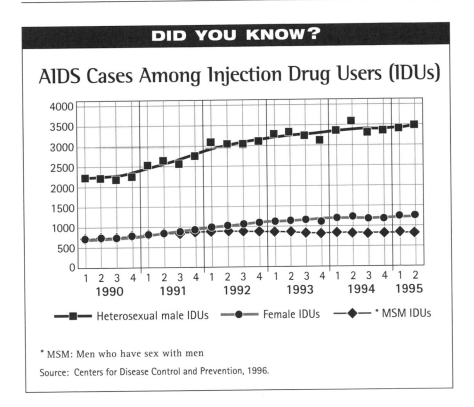

DID YOU KNOW?

AIDS Cases Among Injection Drug Users (IDUs)

—■— Heterosexual male IDUs   —●— Female IDUs   —◆— * MSM IDUs

* MSM: Men who have sex with men

Source: Centers for Disease Control and Prevention, 1996.

are active intravenous drug users and an unknown number of these die from fatal drug overdoses.

These numbers are sobering, but there are some signs that the impact of AIDS on the drug injecting community has caused many to rethink their position on sharing needles. A conscious effort by injection drug users to use new or clean needles would significantly decrease the risk of spreading HIV and hepatitis. However, the best way to prevent contracting such diseases is to avoid injection drugs altogether.

See also: Drug Use, History of; Drugs and Disease; Risk Factors and Risk Taking

■ LAW ON DRUGS, THE

Statutes that provide a wide range of penalties for those convicted of possessing or selling drugs. Cities, states, and the federal government all have laws that deal with drugs. These laws can often be confusing. The laws that apply to teens are a good example. Depending upon a person's age and the circumstances under which he or she is charged with a drug crime, a teen may be tried either as a juvenile or as an adult.

LAWS AND LAW ENFORCEMENT

Although governments have long attempted to control the use of drugs, it wasn't until the early 1900s that major legislation changed the patterns of drug use in the United States. In the 1890s, **opiate** addiction was at its peak in the United States, spurred in no small measure by the use of opiates (drugs with both sedative and euphoric qualities) in many **over-the-counter medicines**. The federal government's first attempt to control their use came in 1906 when Congress passed the Pure Food and Drug Act. The law required medicines containing opiates and other drugs such as **cocaine** (a drug derived from the coca plant that increases energy and alertness and elevates confidence) to be identified as such on their labels. Before this time, manufacturers were not required to disclose the contents of their medicines. However, by the early 1900s the addictive qualities of opiates were becoming apparent to health professionals and the nation at large. The Pure Drug and Food Act of 1906 was a way to check the uncontrolled use of these drugs. The law appeared to have some success in reducing drug addiction in the United States. Congress, however, was not satisfied with a modest reduction in drug use and soon introduced significant changes to the law.

The Harrison Narcotic Act, passed in 1914, prohibited the production and sale of opiates. The law required that cocaine and **heroin** (a drug derived from the Asian poppy that causes drowsiness, relieves pain, and produces euphoria) be used only under the control of a physician, a major change at the time. Cocaine had become an integral part of everyday life; it was even used to make Coca-Cola. When the Harrison Narcotics Act banned its use, the company had to find another substance to give its drink the "kick" that the cocaine had previously provided. The substance the company substituted for cocaine was caffeine, another strong (but legal) stimulant.

Although the intent of the 1914 law was sound, an unexpected backlash occurred. With narcotics now illegal, substitutes began to appear. These substitutes proved to be dangerous due to mislabeling and contamination. By criminalizing the use of drugs, the act also served to brand those addicted to drugs as criminals, rather than people with a medical problem.

The Harrison Narcotic Act was followed in 1920 by a law had an even greater impact on substance abuse in the United States. The law was called the National Prohibition Act, but was more widely known as the Volstead Act, after Andrew Volstead, the congressman who introduced the legislation. Passage of the Volstead Act ushered in a period known as Prohibition, a time when it was a crime to manufacture, distribute, possess, or consume alcohol in the United States. During Prohibition, bars, taverns, and night clubs flourished despite the law. Smuggling became a major source of revenue for organized crime. Gang violence in major cities made figures such as the lawman Elliot Ness and the gangster Al Capone celebrities.

Despite their best efforts, federal law enforcement officials failed to eliminate not only smuggling but also the manufacture of alcohol. The law was unpopular and many people found many ways to get around it. As a result, a number of critics noted a general decline in respect for law and law enforcement. Another unintended result of the law was the rise of organized crime, which prospered as a result of the demand for alcoholic beverages.

In 1933, Congress repealed Prohibition and the use of alcohol was once again legal. The end of Prohibition did not stop the government's campaign against drugs. From 1914 to 1970, Congress enacted 55 laws to address the production, distribution, sale, and use of drugs.

Despite this, the 1970s were a time of increasing drug use in the United States both by teens and adults. Teen use of **marijuana**, cocaine, and other illegal drugs reached historic levels. By the 1980s, concern about the dangerous effects of drug use was mounting in the United States. Before long, Congress passed a new statute, the Anti-Drug Abuse Act of 1986.

The act had a dramatic effect on sentences for drug offenses. The sentence for a first-time offender of a drug crime involving 100 plants or 100 kilograms (220 pounds) of marijuana could be five years in prison. If the amount of marijuana increased to 1,000 plants or 1,000 kilograms (2,200 pounds), the sentence jumped to 10 years. Those who sold five grams (.175 ounces) of **crack** cocaine (equivalent to a couple hundred dollars) could receive a five-year prison sentence with no parole. The sale of 50 grams (1.75 ounces) of cocaine might result in a 10-year sentence. For use of **LSD**, the penalty was enforced if a person sold a single gram (.035 ounces).

Despite the nation's concern about drugs, the law had few supporters among experts in the health field. The experts believed that the law

Drug Schedules

The Controlled Substances Act, part of the 1970 Comprehensive Drug Abuse Prevention and Control, outlines the laws regarding drug enforcement in the United States. The act places all drugs into one of five schedules, based on its medical use and potential for abuse.

SCHEDULE 1

A: Drug has no current accepted medical use.

B: Drug has a high potential for abuse.

Examples: heroin, methaqualone, LSD, peyote, Psilocybin, marijuana, hashish, hash oil, and various amphetamine variants.

SCHEDULE 11

A: Drug has current accepted medical use.

B: Drug has high potential for abuse.

Examples: Dilaudid, Demerol, methadone, cocaine, PCP, morphine and certain cannabis, amphetamine, and barbiturates types.

SCHEDULE 111

A: Drug has current accepted medical use.

B: Drug has medium potential for abuse.

Examples: opium, Vicodin, Tylenol w/codeine and other narcotic, amphetamine, and barbiturate types.

SCHEDULE IV

A: Drug has current accepted medical use.

B: Drug has low potential for abuse.

Examples: Darvocet, Xanax, Valium, Halcyon, Ambien, Ativan, and other barbiturate types.

SCHEDULE V

A: Drug has accepted medical use.

B: Drug has lowest potential for abuse.

Examples: Lomotil, Phenergan, and liquid suspensions.

Source: U.S. Drug Enforcement Agency, 1970.

would not have the intended effect of squeezing the major drug traffickers, but rather would place unreasonable sentences on the small-
time dealers selling on the street. Many felt that the law was far too
harsh, imposing penalties for drug possession and sale that were often
stiffer than those for violent crimes such as assault or armed robbery.

Dissatisfaction led to the Anti-Drug Law of 1988. It was even harsher
than the earlier law. The new law made anyone involved in any aspect
of a drug operation liable for the same punishment as the dealer. As a
result, the lowest person in the operation received the same prison term
as the most important. Although intended to snag high-level figures
involved in drug **trafficking**, the law imprisoned everyone involved in
the drug trade. On the surface, this may seem like a reasonable way to
reduce drug traffic. However, within a six-year period, the law resulted
in a 300 percent increase in the number of prisoners convicted of drug
offenses and a 450 percent increase between 1986 and 1998.

ENFORCEMENT COSTS

Enforcing the drug laws takes an incredible amount of people and
money. The number of government agencies charged with some
aspect of enforcing drug laws is staggering. The Federal Drug Seizure
System (FDSS) involves the Federal Bureau of Investigation (FBI),
Drug Enforcement Agency (DEA), U.S. Border Patrol, U.S. Customs
Service, and U.S. Coast Guard. However, many statewide and local
agencies are also key players in stopping illicit drugs.

- Between 1975 and 2000, 14,560 illegal drug
  laboratories were seized.
- In 2000, 1,901 labs were seized, with 98 percent of them
  manufacturing **methamphetamines**.
- In 2000, the DEA destroyed 2.8 million marijuana
  plants in 40,929 plots, made 9,439 arrests, and seized
  3,463 weapons as well as assets valued at $19.3 million.

Enforcing drug laws is expensive to say the least, but the financial
burden is offset by a practice called **forfeiture**. Forfeiture allows the
government to seize property, cash, boats, airplanes, and virtually
anything else of value that has been used in a drug crime or is purchased with the profits from drug crimes. The seized property is sold
and the proceeds are divided among the law enforcement agencies
that made the bust. This practice has resulted in millions of dollars
being channeled back to cover agency expenses.

Fact Or Fiction?

Forfeiture laws penalize drug kingpins more than small-time users.

Fact: Not true, according to the DEA. In 1991, 83 percent of the total seizures made by law enforcement agencies involved less than $50,000 worth of assets. In addition, 80 percent of all assets seized were taken from suspects who were never charged with any crime.

Some critics of the system fear that overzealous agents may accuse innocent citizens of drug crimes in order to seize their assets. Media outlets including *USA Today* and the television program *60 Minutes* have featured stories about forfeitures based on false accusations. The lack of federal oversight into the way seized assets are being used also worries some observers. The growing number of American citizens falsely accused of profiting from drugs—and having their property and cash seized—has caused concern that basic rights are being violated.

LEGAL COSTS

An unintended consequence of harsher drug laws was an increase in the time, effort, and money needed to enforce these laws. As arrests for drug crimes rose, so has the need for more law enforcement officers and demands placed on the nation's courts and prisons.

Apprehension

The FBI reports that arrests for drug abuse violations by teens 18 years of age and under decreased slightly from 2000 to 2001. However, adult violations increased slightly over the same period. Overall, drug abuse violations have increased 4 percent from 1987 to 2001, according to the FBI.

Of the 13.7 million arrests made by the FBI in 2001, the single largest category was for drug abuse violations. Roughly 1.6 million arrests were made nationwide for drug abuse violations, followed by approximately 1.4 million for DUI (driving under the influence of drugs). The FBI statistics also show that, between 1987 and 1995, heroin and cocaine were the drugs involved in the majority of arrests. Marijuana arrests have exceeded arrests for all other types of drugs.

Prosecution

According to the Bureau of Justice Statistics, in 2001 almost 40,000 suspected drug offenders were prosecuted by the U.S. Attorneys' offices. The figures included those charged with marijuana-related offenses (31 percent), cocaine-related offenses (28 percent), cocaine powder–related offenses (15 percent), and crack cocaine–related offenses (15 percent). Of those offenders arrested for drug violations in 1999, 65 percent had prior drug arrests and 28 percent had five or more prior arrests.

From 1981 to 2000, federal prosecutions of drug defendants increased from less than 20 percent of all crimes to 37 percent. During that same time, the number of suspects prosecuted for drug offenses increased from 8,077 to 28,381. The most frequently tried cases prosecuted in U.S. district courts were those involving drug offenders.

If someone is found guilty in a drug case, the judge is required to hand down the mandatory (fixed) minimum sentence with one exception. If a drug offender provides "substantial assistance" to the Department of Justice—information that assists in the prosecution of other drug offenders—the judge may provide a more lenient sentence. Through this method, the Department of Justice can acquire testimony needed to convict other drug dealers.

However, the practice of using one drug dealer's story against another drug dealer has come under fire due to the inability to confirm the credibility of the testimony. An accused drug dealer has little to lose by providing information to help convict another dealer and he has much to gain—a lighter sentence. There seems to be little that can be done to prevent a drug dealer from fabricating a story simply to reduce his sentence. Despite potential abuses of the law, the federal government still relies on the practice of substantial assistance.

Q & A

Question: What is the most frequently prosecuted offense in U.S. District Court?

Answer: Of all the cases prosecuted before U.S. District Court judges, the most frequently tried cases were those involving drug offenders. From 1981 to 2000, federal prosecutions of drug defendants increased from less than 20 percent of all crimes to 37 percent.

Incarceration

According to a Bureau of Justice Statistics report titled "Federal Criminal Case Processing: 2001," from 1988 to 2001, the number of drug offenders sentenced to prison increased from 79 percent to 90 percent. Over the same time period, the proportion of defendants sentenced to prison for other crimes rose from 54 percent to 74 percent. These numbers show that a person's chance of spending time in prison is much higher if he or she is convicted of a drug crime than with any other type of crime.

Not only were a higher percentage of drug offenders going to prison, but they were also staying longer. The average prison sentence for a drug offense increased from 71.3 months in 1988 to 73.9 months in 2001. Offenders who were involved with crack cocaine, possessed a firearm, or had extensive prior records received the longest prison terms.

The court system refers to people under 18 years of age as juveniles, and in most cases it applies a different set of standards for juvenile offenders than it does for adult offenders. For example, an adult convicted of a **felony** such as dealing large amounts of cocaine must be sentenced to time in prison. A juvenile convicted of the same offense is sent to a youth detention facility or drug rehabilitation program, and the offense typically is erased from his record at age 18. However, in exceptional cases a teen under 18 may be tried as an adult; these situations are called **delinquency cases.**

In 1997, an estimated 1,755,100 delinquency cases were processed in juvenile court. From 1988 to 1997, the number of delinquency cases increased by 48 percent; during the same period, drug law violation cases increased by 125 percent. Teens in general are often involved in drug-related cases. The statistics suggest that younger teens are becoming increasingly involved. According to the Office of Juvenile Justice and Delinquency Prevention, in 1997 teens under the age of 16 were responsible for 40 percent of drug law violation cases.

PUNISHMENT

As a result of the government's strong antidrug policies and mandatory sentencing laws, prison sentences for drug-related crimes receive harsher sentences than other crimes. In 1988, the average prison sentence for persons convicted of drug trafficking averaged 4.5 years, but this turned out to be less than two years in actual time served. Among those convicted of drug possession in 1988, 36 percent were sentenced to city or county jails, 29 percent were sent to state or federal prisons, and 35 percent received probation. The average prison sentence for possession was two years and 11 months, of which the average time served was estimated at 14 months.

Tougher drug laws have placed increasing strains on law enforcement, the courts, and prisons, and on the larger society. As police devote more resources to drug arrests, they have fewer to employ in stopping other types of crime. The nation's courts are becoming overcrowded with drug cases, causing backlogs and delays in the justice system. Yet despite the fact that the federal government and many state governments have spent record amounts on prison construction since the 1980s, overpopulation is still a significant problem.

Despite increasing numbers of drug-related arrests and a rapidly rising prison population, there is no solid evidence that tougher laws are working. Supporters of tougher laws claim that the threat of increased jail time will discourage many people who don't use drugs from trying them in the first place. Opponents of the laws point out that stiffer sentences have not resulted in significant or consistent declines in the use of illegal drugs. They also argue that because there are so many factors that contribute to drug use, it is extremely difficult to determine the impact of any single factor, such as tougher drug laws. The debate is unlikely to be settled any time soon.

See also: Families, Communities, and Drug Abuse

FURTHER READING

Cohen, Peter J. *Drugs, Addiction, and the Law: Policy, Politics, and Public Health.* Durham, NC: Carolina Academic Press, 2004.
Grosshandler, Janet and Ruth C. Rosen (ed.) *Drugs and the Law.* New York: Rosen Publishing Group, 1996.
Miller, Gary J. *Drugs and the Law: Detection, Recognition, and Investigation.* Longwood, FL: Gould Publications, 1997.

■ MEDIA MESSAGES AND COUNTERADVERTISING CAMPAIGNS

Messages about drugs and alcohol communicated through the media—television, film, music, and print sources. Counteradvertising campaigns are messages that challenge positive media images of drugs. The media exercise a powerful influence over the attitudes and behaviors of teens. When it comes to media messages about drugs, that influence can be positive or negative. While some groups use media to warn teens of the dangers of drug use, the media often show drug use as cool or glamorous. Therefore teens need to understand how the media influences their choices about drug use.

TV AND MOVIES

To say that watching movies is a popular pastime with teens would be an understatement. A 1999 study by the Office of National Drug Control Policy reported that teens account for 26 percent of all movie admissions although they make up only 16 percent of the population.

Fact Or Fiction?

Rock lyrics contain more references to drugs than movies do.

Fact: A 1999 study by the Office of National Drug Control Policy and the Department of Health and Human Services found that 98 percent of movies showed illegal drugs, alcohol, tobacco, or over-the-counter/prescription medicines. By contrast, only about 27 percent of the songs studied contained references to drugs.

What connection does going to movies have with drugs? Are movies providing negative drug messages to teens? The study by the Office of National Drug Control Policy found illegal drugs, alcohol, tobacco, or over-the-counter medicines were depicted in 98 percent of the films it examined. These substances were used by the major characters in the film. Five percent of the primary actors used illegal drugs, 25 percent smoked tobacco, and 65 percent consumed alcohol.

When popular movie stars use drugs or alcohol as part of their movie role, they tend to trivialize, normalize, and glorify drug use. Teens are more likely to view these behaviors as acceptable. It's difficult sometimes to remember that it's just a movie and that the actors are simply playing roles.

TV is equally popular with teens. The primary difference is that on TV the promotion of products through advertising is more recognizable. Companies promote their products in movies by having a character use the product; on TV a product is promoted primarily through commercials.

For commercials to be effective, television advertisers need to promote an emotional connection between the product and viewers. That emotional connection is so important that companies pay celebrities handsomely to endorse their products. They reason that if viewers have a positive feeling about a celebrity, that positive feeling may be transferred to the product. If you like Britney Spears or Dale Earnhardt Jr., you will probably consider trying the products they endorse.

Advertisers also try to make an emotional connection with viewers through the use of humor. Many beer commercials use humorous situations or characters to appeal to the viewer. What these advertisements never show, however, is the negative impact alcohol abuse has on the lives of ordinary people. The Centers for Disease Control and Prevention have pointed out that 75 percent of all deaths among 10- to 24-year-olds resulted from just four causes: motor-vehicle crashes, other accidents, homicide, and suicide. Alcohol can be a primary contributor to all four causes, despite the glamorous image of drinking portrayed in beer commercials.

To what extent are decisions about using drugs influenced by advertisements? The truth is that advertising has a greater impact than anyone wants to admit. The American Academy of Pediatrics points out that the average adolescent spends more than 21 hours a week watching television, which means that the typical teen views some 360,000 advertisements before graduating from high school. As a matter of fact, the alcohol industry believes so strongly in the effectiveness of media promotion that it spends $2 billion a year on advertising. So to whom are alcohol companies advertising? This is the million-dollar question. They are adamant that they are not targeting teens with their advertising. Yet their ads show young people using liquor as part of a wide variety of popular activities, including sporting events and parties.

Drug messages are also promoted on TV when popular programs depict the show's stars or other likeable characters abusing alcohol. A 2000 study found that over 75 percent of the episodes of the top 20 TV shows among teens and adults included references to alcohol. Only about one in four episodes that included references to alcohol use mentioned its negative consequences.

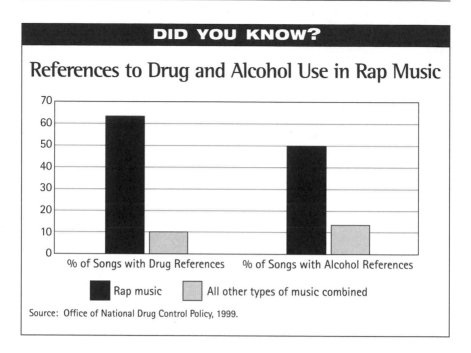

DID YOU KNOW?

References to Drug and Alcohol Use in Rap Music

% of Songs with Drug References   % of Songs with Alcohol References

■ Rap music   ▨ All other types of music combined

Source: Office of National Drug Control Policy, 1999.

MUSIC AND VIDEOS

Music is an important aspect of a teen's life. The 1999 study by the Office of National Drug Policy Control estimates that teens are exposed to music four to six hours per day. Think about the times when you have music playing in the background, while in the car, or doing homework, and it's easy to see where those four to six hours come from.

According to that same study, 35 percent of the songs surveyed contain references to drugs or drug use. However, only 6 percent of the songs containing lyrics about illegal drugs include an anti-use message, and only 3 percent of the songs that referred to alcohol did so. The study did find that music lyrics tended to view the consequences of drug use slightly more unfavorably than favorably. However, the number and nature of references to drug use and its consequences varies according to the type of music a teenager listens to. Rap music, for example, is much more likely to contain lyrics that mention drug use.

COMPUTER GAMES

Computer games have become a mainstay in many teenagers' lives in recent years. According to an article in *New Media Age*, over 40 percent of all TV households had a video game console unit in 1995. Six years later in 2001, Forrester Research estimated that number would climb to 70 percent by 2005. Teenagers spend approximately 4.2 hours per week playing games, primarily at home. Video games are a $7 billion business in the United States.

Critics have noted that in many video games, the main character is repeatedly shown using alcohol or illicit drugs. The effect is to legitimize those behaviors. Over time, teens are likely to forget that the game is a fantasy. They may come to see drug use as acceptable because they tend to view the behaviors exhibited by the characters in video games as normal.

INTERNET

The Internet can be an incredible source of information on virtually any subject. So it comes as no surprise that the Internet is also a source for all kinds of information on illegal drugs. A 2001 study reported in the *American Journal of Psychiatry* found some 81 hallucinogen-related Web sites using just one popular search engine. So how can the Internet promote drug use? Although the Internet is packed with information, not all of it is accurate and some of it is dangerous. The Internet is very similar to other sources of information with one exception—its speed. What might take hours to find in a conventional library is available within seconds on the Internet.

Just as information in books can be misleading, so can information on the Internet. Remember that anyone can post something on the Web, so the quality of Web information needs to be evaluated for accuracy.

Q & A

Question: Where can a teen go for accurate information on drugs?

Answer: If someone tells you that certain substances are "safe," you can check credible Web sites for information, including:

- American Academy of Pediatrics—www.aap.org
- Center for Substance Abuse Prevention—www.forreal.org
- Centers for Disease Control and Prevention—www.cdc.gov
- Clubdrugs.org—www.clubdrugs.org

- Drug Free America—www.drugfreeamerica.org
- National Institute for Drug Abuse—www.nida.nih.gov
- Prevline—www.health.org

Information from the Internet should be read with caution and not relied on until it can be confirmed. Even if the information is accurate, it may still be dangerous. For example, the article in the *American Journal of Psychiatry* quoted above identified a handful of Internet sites that contain all the information needed to "cook up" illegal drugs. The information on those sites may well be accurate, but creating and using drugs based on that information is not only illegal but also very dangerous.

OVERCOMING THE INFLUENCE OF MEDIA

Media education can be an effective way to better understand and counter the influences of negative media images and messages. Advertisers are experienced at developing influential and effective media messages directed at teens. So what can a teen do to counter negative media and messages? The American Academy of Pediatrics (AAP) recommends that teens understand the following:

- All media messages are constructed; that is, they are designed to achieve a specific purpose.
- Media messages shape our understanding of the world.
- Each individual interprets media messages in his or her own way.
- Mass media has powerful economic implications.

The AAP also specifies that a media-educated person is one who is able to:

- limit use of media;
- make positive media choices;
- select creative alternatives to media consumption;
- develop critical thinking and viewing skills; and
- understand the political, social, economic, and emotional implications of all forms of media.

Media education provides a way for teens to be less vulnerable to influences from the media industry. The more teens understand about how media messages are designed and produced, the better prepared they are to make educated decisions for themselves—decisions based on sound information rather than on corporate influence and pressure.

See also: Drugs and Drinking

FURTHER READING

Roberts, Donald F. and Peter G. Christenson. *Here's Looking at You, Kid: Alcohol, Drugs, and Tobacco in Entertainment Media.* Menlo Park, CA: The Henry J. Kaiser Family Foundation, 2000.
Roberts, Donald F., Lisa Henriksen and Peter G. Christenson. *Substance Use in Popular Movies and Music.* Washington, DC: National Drug Control Policy and Department of Health and Human Services, 1999.

▉ MORBIDITY AND MORTALITY

Morbidity, the frequency of illness or injury caused by a particular substance or action, in this case a particular drug; and mortality, the death rate in a given population as the result of taking drugs. Tracking trends in teen drug abuse can be difficult because of the secrecy that often surrounds illegal drug sales. However, morbidity and mortality figures from a wide range of sources can provide a valuable tool for identifying future issues and trends that may impact drug abuse prevention efforts.

INJURY AND ILLNESS FROM DRUG ABUSE

Statistics on morbidity and mortality from drug abuse can be acquired indirectly by examining drug-related injuries and illnesses identified through the criminal justice and health-care systems. Many of the current statistics on drug abuse morbidity are based on drug tests of teens involved in car crashes and of those incarcerated. Criminal justice sources can also provide valuable drug–related information on a teen's cause of death. Health-care facilities collect valuable information on drug use by teens who have been admitted to their care. Mental health providers—especially those who treat teens for substance abuse—can provide important data as well. Statistics about how the number of teens suffering from injuries and illnesses related to drug abuse can reveal trends in teen behaviors. Identifying and studying these trends can provide helpful information on future patterns of drug use.

Morbidity regarding teen drug abuse is closely tied to specific behaviors. The three leading causes of death among teens—suicide, homicide, and motor vehicle crashes—all have direct ties to alcohol and drug abuse. Drug and alcohol abuse are also closely associated with violent acts such as assault and armed robbery as well as with accidents like drowning.

The Drug Abuse Warning Network (DAWN)—a nationwide project of the Office of Applied Studies and the Substance Abuse and Mental Health Services Administration (SAMHSA)—provides data drawn from a survey of 466 hospital emergency departments in 21 metropolitan areas in the United States. DAWN reported an estimated 601,776 drug-related emergency department episodes in 2000. The survey also indicated that between 1999 and 2000, the number of drug-related emergency episodes among teens ages 12–17 rose by 20 percent.

Drug use is related not only to accidents but also to violent behavior. Teens who reported participating in one or more acts of violence during the preceding year were also more likely to use alcohol and illegal drugs. A study reported in 2001 by the Department of Health and Human Services found that 85 percent of teens used **marijuana** (illicit drug that depresses mood and distorts the way the user experiences sights, sounds, and other senses) and that 55 percent used a combination of illegal drugs. Teens who used drugs reported higher rates for behaviors such as fighting at school or work, gang fights, and attacks on others with the intent of seriously hurting them. In 2003, the Web site www.teenviolence.com reported that 25 percent of all teen violence occurs when teens are under the influence of alcohol or drugs. The risk of suicide is also higher for teens who reported alcohol or illicit drug use than for teens who did not use these substances.

According to "Monitoring the Future," an annual study conducted by the National Institute on Drug Abuse (NIDA), teen drug use dropped in 2003 in contrast to previous years for virtually all drugs except **cocaine** and **sedatives**. With this information, treatment professionals and educators are able to focus their efforts on combating the use of these drugs. Data from drug surveys can also help identify increases in teen use of certain drugs or the appearance of new drugs. By identifying a trend quickly, professionals can prepare effective treatment programs and spread the word of the dangers of drug use through a variety of educational outlets.

DEATH RATES

The number of people who died as a consequence of alcohol and drug problems exceeded 132,000 in 1992, with 107,400 of those deaths associated with alcohol abuse and 25,500 associated with drug abuse. However, death rates from drug overdose for teens are extremely low. The majority of the alcohol and drug abuse–related deaths were in the 20 to 40 age group, because the major causes of death, such as motor vehicle crashes, other causes of traumatic death, and HIV infection, are concentrated among this age group. The single largest death rate for teens is from alcohol-related motor vehicle crashes.

CAUSES OF DEATH

DAWN reports mortality data for major cities across the country. Its studies reveal that drug abuse deaths are relatively rare (less than 20 percent of all deaths) for those under age 25. In over half of the cities surveyed by DAWN, the rate of death from drug abuse was less than 10 percent. However statistics for those over the age of 45 are very different, with the rate of drug abuse deaths between 33 percent and 50 percent. DAWN also noted that in the average metropolitan area roughly 50 percent of drug abuse deaths were ruled accidental, 17 percent suicides, and 30 percent due to undetermined or other causes. Drug abuse deaths rarely occur from the use of a single drug. The use of multiple drugs was reported in the overwhelming majority of drug abuse deaths across the country. Some 90 percent of drug abuse

---

DID YOU KNOW?

Number of Deaths Attributed to Drug Abuse, 1992–1998

Data Series	1992	1993	1994	1995	1996	1997	1998
Deaths Attributable to Drug Abuse	24,476	24,206	26,234	26,823	23,283	19,268	19,277

Source: The Lewin Group, 2001.

deaths involving **heroin** also included another drug, and almost 80 percent of deaths involving cocaine included another, as well. Research has shown that three specific drugs are used most frequently when a combination of drugs result in death. Those three drugs are heroin, cocaine, and alcohol. All three have profound physical effects on the heart, central nervous system, and pulmonary system (the system that distributes oxygen throughout the body). When these substances are used together, their physical effects can be lethal.

The DAWN study also reported on deaths from abuse of prescription and over-the-counter drugs. Two classes of **prescription drugs**—benzodiazepines and narcotic analgesics—were responsible for most of the deaths attributed to prescription drugs. The benzodiazepines, which include Valium and Librium, are a family of drugs prescribed to combat anxiety. Narcotic analgesics, drugs prescribed for pain relief, include methadone, codeine, hydrocodone, oxycodone, and diphenhydramine.

POPULATIONS MOST AFFECTED

The population most affected by alcohol and drug abuse depends on the specific drug. Males, for example, are significantly more likely than females to be involved in motor-vehicle crashes involving alcohol or drug use. Females, on the other hand, are more likely to attempt suicide, a behavior frequently associated with drug and alcohol abuse. The use of inhalants is most likely to involve younger teens from lower socioeconomic groups. Female teens are more likely than their male peers to report that cocaine, crack, **LSD**, and heroin were easy to obtain.

For all teens, involvement in suicide, homicide, violence, or motor-vehicle crashes probably have some ties to alcohol and drug abuse, according to the 2000 DAWN survey. The message is clear: abusing alcohol or drugs increases the chances of illness, injury, or death regardless of ethnicity, place of residence, or socioeconomic background. Perhaps the single most effective thing one can do to increase the chances of leading a long, healthy life is to avoid drugs and alcohol.

See also: Crack Cocaine; Depression and Drugs; Driving Under the Influence of Drugs; Drugs and Criminal Activity; Drugs and Disease; Illegal Drugs, Common; Inhalants; Media Messages and Counteradvertising Campaigns; Over-the-Counter Drugs

■ OVER-THE-COUNTER DRUGS

Legal medications that can be purchased without a prescription from a medical professional. Over-the-counter (OTC) drugs include commonly available pain medications such as aspirin, acetaminophen (Tylenol), and ibuprofen (Advil); cold and flu remedies; laxatives; and a wide range of other substances. A related class of drugs are **prescription drugs**, which are also legal but may only be acquired with a prescription from a doctor. Even though they are legal, misuse of prescription and OTC drugs can lead to both **psychological dependence** (reliance on a substance for normal functioning) and **physical dependence** (intense craving for a drug that is not accompanied by physical dependence). People may increase their intake of these drugs to ensure a sense of well-being while treated for unrelated illnesses or health problems. They may also engage in nonmedical use of OTC or prescription drugs. Regardless of the reason, abuse of OTC and prescription drugs is both dangerous and illegal.

COMMONLY ABUSED OVER-THE-COUNTER DRUGS

OTC medications can be divided into several different categories: **stimulants**, analgesics, and cough and cold medications. This article lists a large number of common OTC drugs, but it's important to remember that, with new drugs coming on the market all the time, no list can ever be completely accurate. In addition, virtually any medication can be abused, so just because a drug doesn't appear in the list, doesn't mean it can't be abused.

The OTC stimulants are divided into two types of drugs: **amphetamines** and caffeine. Diet pills contain amphetamines, while caffeine is found in a wide array of products including coffee, tea, many soft drinks, pain medications, and allergy and cold remedies. Both amphetamines and caffeine are used to delay the onset of mental and physical fatigue. Because they increase short-term energy, they are often abused by people who work long hours or athletes looking for a physical advantage in their sport.

Consuming excessive doses of stimulants over an extended period of time may lead to anxiety, **hallucinations**, severe **depression**, or physical and psychological dependence. Teens need to be aware that stimulants are in a wide variety of everyday products. Checking labels is important.

Analgesics are OTC drugs that typically are used to treat fever, pain, and arthritis. The most common analgesic is aspirin; other widely available analgesics include acetaminophen and ibuprofen.

Possible side effects of taking too much aspirin include nausea, heartburn, or the development of bleeding ulcers. To reduce the possibility of these side effects, aspirin can be purchased in a coated form. Acetaminophen, which is the active ingredient in Tylenol, is also used to treat aches, pains and fevers. However, unlike aspirin, it is usually free from side effects. Large doses, however, may cause rashes, fevers, or changes in blood composition. Ibuprofen, which is sold under such brand names as Motrin, Advil, and Nuprin, is used to relieve discomfort associated with arthritis, menstrual cramping, fever, and muscle strains. Side effects such as upset stomach, dizziness, drowsiness, headache, or ringing in the ears may occur. Abuse of this OTC drug may lead to confusion, tingling in hands and feet, and vomiting.

Q & A

Question: Can a teen die from an overdose of aspirin?

Answer: Yes, but it is rare. Aspirin is an analgesic. As one of the three most popular analgesics, aspirin—along with acetaminophen, and ibuprofen—is widely used to treat fever, arthritis and pain. The signs and symptoms of aspirin overdose can include hyperactivity, fever, convulsions, collapse, low blood pressure, rapid heart rate, rapid breathing, and, possibly, respiratory failure. Aspirin overdose can also produce wheezing, ringing in the ears, deafness, nausea and vomiting, dry mouth, bleeding, dizziness, hallucinations, and drowsiness. The best advice in the event of aspirin overdose is to call poison control or the local hospital emergency room. The following procedures may be performed, depending on the severity of the situation:

- Gastric lavage (stomach pump)
- Administration of activated charcoal to neutralize salicylic acid, the active ingredient in aspirin
- Administration of a laxative to flush the aspirin from the victim's body
- Taking of a blood sample to determine the salicylate level in blood and arterial blood gasses
- Administration of fluids (milk, fruit juices or, in severe cases, IV fluids) to prevent dehydration
- Administration of a sponge bath to control fever
- Administration of medications as needed

Most cold preparations are designed to treat specific cold symptoms and provide temporary relief from discomfort. There are several categories of commonly used cold remedies. Antihistamines are typically used to relieve the itchy, watery eyes caused by allergies or cold and flu viruses. As their name suggests, decongestants are intended to reduce congestion of the sinuses, nose, and throat due to allergies, colds, and flu. Both antihistamines and decongestants can cause drowsiness or excitability. Antitussives are cough suppressants used to treat painful, persistent coughs. Expectorants are used to help clear mucous from the respiratory system. Both of these types of medications may contain alcohol and some may contain analgesic narcotics, such as codeine, to relieve pain and induce sleep. They may be **addictive**.

Fact Or Fiction?

The most widely abused category of over-the-counter drugs is laxatives.

Fact: Laxatives are the most widely misused and abused of all over-the-counter medications. Laxatives are primarily intended for short-term use to ease constipation; however, excessive and continual use overtime can lead to dependency. Any drug that creates dependency can affect a teen both psychologically and physically.

COMMONLY ABUSED PRESCRIPTION DRUGS

Prescription drugs make complex surgery possible, relieve temporary pain for millions of people, and enable many individuals with chronic (long-term) medical conditions to control their symptoms and lead productive lives. Most people who take prescription medications use them responsibly. However, the nonmedical use of prescription drugs can lead to abuse and addiction, characterized by compulsive drug use.

Antidepressants

Antidepressants are prescription medications used to treat depression, a disease affecting over 15 million Americans. Some of the original antidepressants were Nardil, Tofranil and Elavil. Although not technically an antidepressant, lithium, which is used to treat **bipolar disorder,** is often included in this group. The side effects of prolonged and excessive use of these drugs include excessive urination or thirst, diarrhea, vomiting, drowsiness, dizziness, or muscle weakness. Some newer antidepressants are Wellbutrin, Prozac, and Zoloft. There are fewer side effects with these medications. In 2004 the U.S. Food and Drug Administration advised that antidepressants prescribed to children might initially worsen depression and increase the risk of suicide and called for warning labels and further investigation, particularly into the possibility of similar effects in adults.

Sedatives and tranquilizers
Sedatives are drugs prescribed to encourage sleep, while tranquilizers are commonly used to treat anxiety. A family of drugs called benzodiazepines, which include Valium and Librium, are the most widely prescribed tranquilizers and sleep-inducing medications. Other drugs used to treat anxiety and tension are Xanax, Ativan, and Tranxene. Common sleeping medications include Dalamine, Restotril and Halcion. Possible side effects of these drugs include drowsiness, poor coordination, and light-headedness.

Overuse of sedatives and tranquilizers can lead to respiratory difficulties, sleeplessness, coma, and even death. Seconal, Phenopbarbital, and Nembutal are less commonly prescribed medications used to treat anxiety and insomnia. If improperly used, these drugs can cause an individual to feel depressed or experience respiratory difficulties.

MISUSE AND DEPENDENCE
Over $78 billion in prescription and OTC drugs are produced each year in the United States. According to the Substance Abuse and Mental Health Services Administration (SAMHSA), OTC and prescription drug abusers made up only 3 percent of the 1.6 million admissions reported to the Treatment Episode Data Set (TEDS) in 1999. TEDS tracks admissions to and releases from facilities that treat people for abuse of alcohol and drugs. SAMHSA also reports that OTC medications made up only 2 percent of the 44,000 treatment admissions in 1999, with the remaining number being tied to prescription drug abuse. Considering the sheer number of OTC drugs, the rate of abuse is low.

In 1998, the SAMHSA National Household Survey on Drug Abuse showed that more than 20 million people over the age of 12 reported using one or more psychotherapeutic drugs (stimulants, sedatives, tranquilizers, and analgesics available through prescription) for nonmedical purposes at some time in their lives. Stimulants, analgesics,

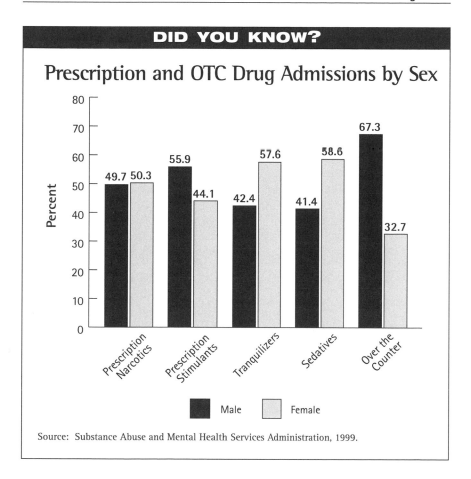

DID YOU KNOW?

Prescription and OTC Drug Admissions by Sex

Source: Substance Abuse and Mental Health Services Administration, 1999.

and tranquilizers were the most widely used drugs that fit this category. Nearly half (46 percent) of the 44,000 treatment admissions for primary prescription and OTC drug abuse in 1999 were for prescription narcotic drugs. Prescription stimulant drugs accounted for an additional 33 percent of admissions, while tranquilizers accounted for 11 percent. Sedatives and OTC medications made up 7 percent and 2 percent of these admissions, respectively.

Addiction rarely occurs among people who use pain relievers, central nervous system depressants, or stimulants as prescribed. However, inappropriate use of prescription drugs can lead to addiction. In addition, the amphetamines found in many diet pills have been tied to the development of anorexia nervosa, a disease associated with extreme dieting and excessive thinness.

Many medications contain alcohol or sedative drugs such as codeine, which can be addictive and life threatening. Young people may abuse these medications for the effects derived from alcohol use, as the alcohol content in some OTC preparations may be as high as 40 percent. In addition, the use of alcohol, a depressant, with some prescription and OTC drugs may inhibit or enhance the drug's effectiveness and cause a loss of coordination. Combining OTC drugs with some prescription drugs can cause similar effects or even more harmful types of reactions.

Patients, health-care professionals, and pharmacists all have roles in preventing misuse and addiction. For example, physicians and other health-care providers should screen patients for substance abuse during routine history-taking by asking questions about what prescriptions and OTC medicines the patient is taking and why. If a doctor prescribes a pain medication, central nervous system depressant, or stimulant, the patient should follow the directions for use carefully. He or she should also learn what effects the drug may have and the impact of interactions with other drugs by reading all information provided by the pharmacist. The pharmacist should make sure the patient understands how to use the medication and answer any questions about its use.

See also: Drug Abuse, Causes of; Drugs and Drinking

FURTHER READING
Brodin, Michael. *The Over-the-counter Drug Book.* New York: Pocket Books, 1998.
Leber, Max, Max R. Leger, Anthony Scalzo, et al. *The Handbook of Over-the-counter Drugs and Pharmacy Products.* Berkeley, CA: Celestial Arts, 2000.
Reader's Digest. *Prescription and Over-the-counter Drugs.* Pleasantville, NY: Reader's Digest, 2001.

■ OVERDOSE AND DRUGS

The accidental or intentional use of a drug or medicine in an amount high enough to cause an adverse physical reaction. Virtually any substance, from **over-the-counter drugs** to **prescription drugs** to illegal drugs, can be abused and thus result in overdose. Many drugs, when combined with other substances, taken with alcohol, or taken in amounts beyond the recommended dose, can lead to an overdose. Certain groups are at a greater risk for overdose, including children and people coping with suicidal tendencies resulting from depression, a mental disorder characterized by symptoms such as hopelessness and sadness. Teens are at increased risk of an overdose, because suicide is a leading killer of adolescents.

WHAT CAUSES AN OVERDOSE?

Overdose can occur by accident or design. An accidental overdose occurs most frequently among children and the elderly. Young children put almost anything they find in their mouths, including drugs or chemicals. The elderly, on the other hand, typically take a whole battery of drugs on a regular schedule. Many consult a variety of specialists and receive different medications from each of them. Sometimes the combination of certain drugs will cause a reaction different from the one intended. At other times, an elderly person may unintentionally take larger doses of the drugs than prescribed, thus causing an overdose. Drug-tracking systems in pharmacies have helped reduce the problem of drug interactions caused by taking medicines prescribed by different physicians. New devices for assisting visually impaired seniors are also being used to prevent overmedicating.

Accidental overdose also occurs when users of illicit drugs take a combination of drugs with unexpected and sometimes deadly results. Some dealers "cut" or mix their drugs with other substances to increase the volume of the drug so that more can be sold. These dealers will use almost any cutting agent, from crushed aspirin to baking soda. These cutting agents not only distort the effects of the drug, but also impact its potency. Since many illicit drugs are made or cut in underground laboratories, quality control is limited at best and the result is little consistency from one dose to another. A drug that makes someone feel good one time can be disastrous the next. Combining drugs with others or alcohol also can have a deadly impact. For example, both alcohol and barbiturates work by depressing the functions of the circulatory system, which delivers oxygen and nutrients throughout the body and controls respiration. Mixing the two depressants can slow down or stop one's breathing, leading to coma and even death.

The same drug can have greatly varied effects on different people. A particular dose of a drug that may be fine for one person may result in an overdose in someone else. Just as drugs affect different people in different ways, their impact can take longer to appear in some users than in others. A person who takes a drug and does not experience its effects as quickly as expected may become impatient and take another dose before the original dose has had time to produce the desired effects. In many cases, taking the additional amount is enough to cause an overdose.

Not all overdoses are accidental. When a person deliberately takes an excessive amount of drugs with the goal of overdosing, it is called an **intentional overdose**. Intentional overdoses are a common form of suicide, and suicide is a leading cause of death among teens.

RATES

Death from overdose has increased significantly since 1990. A large number of accidental overdoses are attributed to users of injection drugs who mix drugs. However, intentional overdose is also a serious problem among other drug users. A third of all overdose deaths are intentional. Chronic (long-term) drug use can cause increasingly depressed feelings in an individual, thus making the person more likely to attempt an intentional overdose.

DANGERS OF OVERDOSE

The dangers of overdose depend largely upon the kind of drug a person takes. Overdoses of **depressants**—drugs that depress the central nervous system—can be extremely dangerous. This class of drugs includes a wide range of substances including alcohol, **opiates**, and **prescription drugs** such as barbiturates, **tranquilizers**, **antidepressants**, and narcotic analgesics. All of these drugs slow respiration (breathing) and, when taken in large enough doses, can depress breathing to dangerously low levels. Symptoms of overdose from a depressant include slow and shallow breathing, clammy skin, extremely low blood pressure, convulsions, respiratory failure, coma, and possibly death.

Taking a combination of depressants can be particularly lethal. The combined effects of two different depressants can be more powerful than the effects of a single one. Alcohol is probably the depressant most frequently used in combination with other depressants and represents a major cause of overdose. The National Institute on Alcohol Abuse and Alcoholism reported that overdoses involving a combination of alcohol and prescription drugs may have played a part in up to 25 percent of all emergency room visits in 1995.

Stimulants such as **amphetamines** and **methamphetamines** have the opposite effect of depressants, but an overdose of stimulants can be just as deadly. Stimulants increase heart and respiratory rates and elevate blood pressure. Increased dosages of stimulants produce symptoms including rapid or irregular heartbeat, loss of coordination, and physical collapse. Overdose of stimulants can result in blurred vision, dizziness, restlessness, anxiety, **delusions** (false or distorted perceptions), intense agitation, fever, **hallucinations**, **convulsions**, and possible death.

Symptoms of a **cocaine** or **crack** cocaine overdose are similar to those involving a stimulant overdose. They include seizures, high blood pressure, increased heart rate, **paranoia**, and other changes in behavior. Both heart attack and stroke are serious risks within three days of cocaine overdose, a particular issue of concern for those who use crack.

Overdoses of **hallucinogens** such as **LSD** and **PCP**, and **designer drugs** including **ecstasy**, can also have severe consequences. Long-term or chronic use of hallucinogens may cause depression, violent behavior, anxiety, and distorted perceptions of time. An overdose can result in convulsions, **psychosis**, coma, and death.

Recent research has pinpointed the dangers associated with overdoses of a category of drugs known as anabolic steroids. Steroids are synthetic compounds that are used to improve athletic performance by increasing body weight and muscle strength. Steroids offer the temptation of quick results. While the use of steroids may cause quick weight and muscle gains, it can also generate mood swings and extremely aggressive behavior typically called "roid rage." An overdose also results in severe skin rashes and impotence in males. An overdose in females may result in the development of irreversible masculine traits, such as increased facial hair and interrupted menstruation.

Even over-the-counter drugs can be dangerous when used to excess. An overdose of acetaminophen (Tylenol) can cause liver damage. In the initial stages of overdose, symptoms include loss of appetite, tiredness, nausea and vomiting, paleness, and sweating. By the final stage of liver failure, the person becomes jaundiced (a yellowing of the skin and whites of the eyes caused by the death of red blood cells).

Aspirin, as well as some muscle and joint creams, can contain substances called salicylates that have the potential for overdose. When used in excess, these substances can produce symptoms that include irritation of the stomach and intestine, fever, and vomiting. Overdoses of salicylates may cause rapid heartbeat, fast breathing, confusion, hallucinations, tiredness, and ringing in the ears. The most serious symptoms are acute renal (kidney) failure, coma, and heart failure.

Marijuana is the illegal drug most widely abused by teens. An overdose is rarely if ever fatal, except when users attempt to drive a car or operate machinery while under the influence of the drug. Symptoms of overdose can include fatigue, lack of coordination, paranoia, and **drug psychosis**.

EMERGENCY RESPONSE AND TREATMENT

Any first responder (police officer, firefighter, or paramedic) to a medical emergency looks for immediate symptoms which may be life threatening. Overdose emergencies are no different. However, the effects of the drug on the victim may make it more difficult for the first responder to do his or her job effectively. For example, if the person is

---

DID YOU KNOW?

Risk of Overdose in Combination with Other Factors

Risks increase when the user:

- mixes drugs and alcohol;
- uses opiates such as heroin while using another drug or drugs;
- uses opiates after a period of **abstinence** when **tolerance** will be low;
- has a history of overdose;
- has a long history of **injection drug** use;
- shares used injection equipment such as needles;
- has a high alcohol intake;
- has a high drug intake;
- has suicidal thoughts;
- has feelings of **depression; and**
- has not been in a treatment program.

Source: Centers for Disease Control and Prevention, 1998.

conscious, he or she can provide key information such as what drugs were ingested and in what quantities. He or she will also be able to inform the first responder if alcohol is involved. However, if the victim is unconscious, the only information available will be from friends and bystanders, who may not know what drug the victim took or may provide inaccurate information. In either case, the first responder may not have all the information needed to properly treat the victim.

Q & A

Question: What information do I need to contact a poison control center about an overdose?

Answer: The information needed by any first responder or poison control center is the same. The information you need to have should include:

- Whether the person is conscious
- Whether the person is breathing
- What drug(s) were taken
- How much of the drug was taken
- When the drug was taken
- Whether the drug was taken with alcohol or any other drugs or chemicals
- The age of the person
- The symptoms the victim is experiencing

A drug overdose can be frightening. It's important to keep your wits about you so that the necessary information can be given to the first responder. Your calmness may mean the difference between life or death.

In case of an overdose, determining what drug was taken and how fast it will be absorbed into the system is critical. Having all of the necessary information at hand is extremely important in helping a first responder successfully treat an overdose.

See also: Depression and Drugs; Drugs and Drinking; Morbidity and Mortality; Over-the-Counter Drugs; Steroids, Anabolic

FURTHER READING

Cohen, Jay S. *Over Dose: The Case against the Drug Companies: Prescription Drugs, Side Effects, and Your Health.* New York: Putnam, 2001.

Graedon, Joe and Teresa Graedon. *Dangerous Drug Interactions.* New York: St. Martin's Press, 1995.

Olsen, Kent R. *Poisoning and Drug Overdose.* Stamford, CT: Appleton and Lange, 1998.

■ PEER PRESSURE AND DRUGS

Influence exerted by one's peers—people of the same age or social group—to act or behave in a certain way. Everyone wants to make friends and get along with people, and teens are especially eager to be accepted by their peers. However, when peers accept or encourage drug and alcohol use, a teen may feel pressure to do the same for fear of being rejected. Such negative peer pressure is a risk factor in teen drug and alcohol abuse. Peers can also be a positive influence on one another by avoiding alcohol and illegal drugs.

EFFECTS OF PEER PRESSURE

In a 2001 survey by the Pew Foundation, 82 percent of Americans named peer pressure as a major factor in determining whether a teen will use illegal drugs. However, some researchers have disputed the connection between peer pressure and teen drug and alcohol use. In 1996, the journal *Addiction* published an article titled "On the Importance of Peer Influence for Adolescent Drug Use: Commonly Neglected Considerations." The article suggested that factors such as family environment, socioeconomic status, and heredity may be as or more important than peer pressure in determining teen behavior. These findings may help explain why school drug programs that focus on resisting peer pressure have not achieved better results.

Other studies, however, do show a relationship between peer behavior and drug use. One conducted in 2001 by the Substance Abuse and Mental Health Services Administration (SAMHSA) suggested that teens who had a few close friends who smoked **marijuana** were 39 times more likely to use the drug than teens whose friends did not smoke. The same study found that teens are 16 times less likely to try marijuana if they think their friends would be "very upset" if they did not do so. Clearly, among the teens surveyed by SAMHSA, peer attitudes made a big difference.

TEENS SPEAK

Kim Seemed Like a Great Person

I'm Pat, and I've been friends with Kim for only a short period of time because I just moved here. I didn't meet Kim until school started, but we became close friends very quickly. She seemed like a great person, popular with the cool girls and guys alike. Kim was always concerned about how I was doing and was so considerate of my feelings, wishes, and interests.

One Friday night, Kim asked me if I wanted to go to the volleyball match at the high school. It sounded like a good time, and I rarely passed up an opportunity to spend time with Kim. At halftime, Kim suggested that we leave and meet up with some other kids from school. I want to emphasize that Kim had never been anything but a super person and good friend. But when we met up with the others, Kim started to act weird, talking trash and trying to be all cool. It became apparent to me that she was trying to impress people by acting "all bad."

As I met different people at the party, one of Kim's friends, who was obviously "wasted," offered me a strange-looking pill and said, "Take one; it's the bomb and everybody's doing it." All of a sudden I got this sick feeling in my stomach just thinking how stupid I was to have befriended this obnoxious person. Not wanting to seem like a nerd, I told Kim's friend that I had been on strong medication to control my anger and aggression and that any other drug could cause me to become very hostile. I figured if I was going to make up something, it might as well be a good story.

I had no interest in doing whatever pill they had, but to save face I provided an alternative reason why I couldn't. Even if I was pressured, I was going to stand my ground. I would have eventually just walked away if I had been pressured at all. Actually, I had planned ahead for such a situation so I was prepared. One thing's for sure—Kim is history.

In 2003, the University of Pennsylvania's Annenberg Public Policy Center published a study that revealed a troubling aspect of the relationship between peer pressure and drug use. The study, "Young Americans Say Alcohol, Marijuana, Cigarettes, and Lottery Tickets are Easily Accessible," found that people between the ages of 14 and 22 are more likely to connect behavior such as drinking, using drugs, smoking cigarettes, and gambling to popular kids rather than unpopular ones.

Researchers are also discovering that peer pressure begins at a younger age than many people suspect. The National Institutes of Health in 2001 reported that peer attitudes may influence a child's decision about smoking and drinking as early as sixth grade. The study found that elementary school children held generally negative attitudes toward smoking and drinking. By middle school, however, young people are more likely to associate with friends who smoke or drink as well as to smoke and drink themselves. Middle-school girls were more likely than boys to be swayed by peer pressure to drink. The study also showed that these behavior patterns tended to remain throughout high school.

Q & A

Question: What are the steps a teen can take to make a good decision?

Answer: Decision making can be difficult at any age. Professionals suggest six steps to making good decisions. They will not help you make a snap decision, but they can be helpful when you have time to go through each step carefully. The steps include:

1. Identify the problem. What decision do you have to make?
2. Consider your values. What is important to you?
3. List the options. What possible actions could you take?
4. Weigh the consequences. List the pros and cons of each option.
5. Decide and act. Describe what you will do. Explain your decision.
6. Evaluate your choice. How do you feel about the action you took? Did you make a good decision? Would you take a different action if faced with the same scenario?

RESISTING PEER PRESSURE

You've probably heard the peer pressure speech from your parents a thousand times, right? The one where they ask, "If so-and-so jumped off a cliff, would you jump off too?" Well, it may seem corny, but it carries an important message about thinking for yourself. It's not easy to resist the pressure to do something your friends are telling you is "cool," even if you know it's not the right thing to do.

Fact Or Fiction?

A teen can fend off anyone who is pressuring him or her to use drugs by using refusal skills.

Fact: Having a prepared refusal response makes it easier to withstand even intense peer pressure. Refusal skills are rehearsed responses to pressure from peers to use drugs. They may include invented stories, bogus instructions from parents, and even the truth. The following are ways to counter the pressure to use drugs without losing face:

- Say no. How would you say no to pressure?
- Offer an alternative. What else could you do with friends?
- Stand your ground. What would you do if friends kept pressuring you?
- Walk away. How would you get out of the situation?
- Plan ahead. What could you do to avoid this situation? Who can help you practice refusing peer pressure?
- Have a support system. Who will stand by you and how can you best use their support?

Recent studies showing a drop in teen drug use suggest that young people are getting better at resisting pressure to use alcohol and drugs. The National Institute on Drug Abuse's 2003 "Monitoring the Future" study shows that teen use of all drugs has steadily declined since the mid-1990s. Some school officials attribute the decline to a combination of parental and neighborhood involvement, as well as positive peer pressure from students to avoid drugs. They report that, compared to 10 years ago, fewer students today think using alcohol or drugs is "cool."

See also: Risk Factors and Risk Taking

FURTHER READING

Donatelle, R.J. and L.G. Davis. *Access to Health,* 5th ed. Needham Heights, MA: Allyn & Bacon Publishing, 1996.

Myers, Arthur. *Drugs and Peer Pressure.* New York: Rosen Publishing Group, 1995.

■ PRENATAL EXPOSURE TO DRUGS

See: Drugs and Development

■ REHABILITATION AND TREATMENT

The process of breaking the physical, mental, and spiritual bonds of addiction to drugs and alcohol and returning to normal functioning. Rehabilitation is most effective when accompanied by a comprehensive, individually designed treatment program. The individually designed program is important because every addiction is different. Individualized programs assist teens in dealing with the issues of greatest concern in their recovery. Comprehensiveness is important because addiction impacts not only the teen's physical, mental, and spiritual well-being but also the lives of family and friends. Overcoming addiction is greatly enhanced by a reputable rehabilitation and treatment program.

WHAT IS INVOLVED IN REHABILITATION?

There are two stages to rehabilitation from drug or alcohol abuse: **detoxification** and recovery. Detoxification is the process of completely removing the drug from one's system. Only after he or she is freed of physical dependence from the drug can the process of recovery begin. Recovery involves learning about the nature of addiction in general as well as about the circumstances surrounding one's own addiction. This knowledge is invaluable in helping one identify harmful influences or patterns of behavior that increase his or her chances of using drugs again. Both detoxification and recovery are necessary to break addiction and return to a normal life.

DETOXIFICATION

Detoxification can take several different forms, depending on the type of addiction, the level of addiction, and the patient's ability to pay.

Because drug addiction withdrawal is difficult, medical support is frequently required. Although some drug users may initiate detoxification themselves (a process known as "going cold turkey"), most require assistance as withdrawal symptoms intensify. Many detoxification programs use substances called agonists and antagonists to block the action of drugs in the nervous system. As a result, even if the patient abuses a drug while in detoxification, the drugs will have no effect. The use of these substances is typically combined with some form of counseling or therapy to bring about behavior changes.

In residential or inpatient detoxification programs, withdrawal from addiction takes place in a supportive and supervised environment. The use of residential detoxification should be considered if:

- The risk of severe withdrawal symptoms, such as epileptic seizures or extreme agitation, is high;
- The home environment is inadequate to support the detoxification and rehabilitation process, or other drug users are present;
- The teen is homeless or is currently residing in a crisis shelter; or
- Previous attempts through nonresidential or community detoxification failed.

Residential or inpatient detoxification can be medically assisted or nonmedical, depending on the situation. Reasons for a medical residential detoxification would include a history of severe withdrawal symptoms, coexisting medical problems such as heart disease, multiple drug and alcohol dependencies, or a previous failures with nonmedical residential detoxification. Nonmedical residential detoxification is appropriate for those who do not have a severe addiction. In such cases, medications are unnecessary and the individual can work through the withdrawal with counseling and support. When the dependency is mild and the individual is sufficiently motivated, nonresidential or outpatient based detoxification may be the best route to take. When drug addiction results in a profound decrease in normal levels of mental and physical functioning, urgent care may be required. Before treatment can be initiated, a medical assessment is necessary to rule out other possible causes of the condition.

A wide variety of detoxification programs exist. Each uses different methods to rid the body of drugs. The most widely advertised form of detoxification is known as rapid, anesthesia-assisted detoxification (RAAD), also called "rapid detoxification" or "ultrarapid detoxification." RAAD, used in cases of **opiate** addiction, is typically a four-to-six hour treatment during which a patient withdraws from addiction while safely asleep under general anesthesia. In newer forms of RAAD the patient receives the drug naltrexone, which blocks the action of opiates in the nervous system. After the procedure, the patient remains hospitalized for approximately 24 hours. This procedure requires professional medical assistance by a licensed physician in a medical facility. RAAD is frequently followed up with counseling and other outpatient services as needed.

With some drugs, the best approach to detoxification is to gradually reduce dosage over a period of time. For example, detoxification for a person taking 30 milligrams of Valium a day might include reducing the dose by 5 milligrams per month. However, for other drugs, such as **cocaine** or **amphetamines**, detoxification can be rapid and abrupt. Rapid detoxification usually results in a strong craving for the drug along with withdrawal symptoms such as depression, anxiety, agitation, and fatigue. These symptoms typically fade in eight to nine days, but in some cases the patient is given drugs such as desipramine to relieve the withdrawal symptoms.

The detoxification programs described here are only a fraction of those available. Some programs encourage dietary changes, while others use holistic therapies that seek to cure addiction by changing many aspects of a person's lifestyle and behavior. The best method is the one that works best for the individual. A call to a family physician, local mental health department, or Alcoholics Anonymous (AA) may yield a list of some local programs with successful track records.

RECOVERY

Once detoxification has been completed, the process of recovery can begin. The first step is for the patient to gain a clearer understanding of his or her addiction. Many treatment programs view addiction as a complex disease that damages the individual not only physically but also mentally and spiritually. Because the disease impacts all three areas, recovery efforts must also go beyond the physical and address emotional and spiritual needs.

Experts disagree over whether addiction is a disease or a learned behavior. Those who view it as a disease regard addiction as similar to other illnesses over which the individual has little control. Those who view addiction as a behavior regard it as a choice. To support the idea of addiction as a disease, recent research suggests there may be a genetic component to addiction. In addition, physiological changes in the brain have been identified that can result from drug use. These two research findings lend credibility to the idea that addiction is a disease and not simply a learned behavior.

Types of therapy

Therapy involves the examination of one's behaviors. It takes hard work to change behaviors associated with drug abuse by talking about them. Most therapists believe that drug abuse disorders are difficult to treat because they often require structure and a multiple treatment approach to be successful. To effectively treat addicted teens, it is important to combine therapy with knowledge of the treatment process, including an understanding of the drug itself as well as its intoxication and withdrawal effects, a working knowledge of drug culture and addictive lifestyles, and knowledge of various recovery programs.

According to Alan Leshner, director of the National Institute on Drug Abuse, therapy that combines a variety of approaches is more effective than a single approach, because addiction is both a biological and a behavioral disorder. Bruce Rounsaville, the principal investigator at two major clinical research centers for the study of substance abuse and psychiatric disorders at Yale University, argues that combining treatments is more effective because different treatments address different aspects of the addiction. Medications such as naltrexone tackle the physiological aspects of addiction, while psychotherapy and counseling explore behavioral issues related to drug use.

One form of psychotherapy used for treating addiction is called cognitive-behavioral therapy, or CBT. This approach focuses on teaching patients how to recognize and avoid situations in which they are likely to use drugs. In addition, CBT aims to help patients control their urge to use drugs and deal with the emotional, psychological, and practical problems caused by their addiction.

Another popular form of therapy, called the 12-Step Program, was pioneered by AA and is now used by many other groups seeking to end an addiction. The 12 steps of the program reflect the basic changes that need to be made for recovery. The steps include:

1. Admitting that you are powerless over the drug and that your life has become unmanageable

2. Believing that a higher spiritual power can restore you to normal functioning

3. Making a decision to turn your will and your life over to the care of God according to your own spiritual beliefs

4. Making a moral inventory of your life

5. Admitting to God, to yourself, and to another human being the exact nature of your wrongs

6. Being ready to have God remove all these defects of character

7. Humbly asking God to remove your shortcomings

8. Making a list of all persons you have harmed, and being willing to make amends to them all

9. Making direct amends to such people wherever possible, except when to do so would injure them or others

10. Continuing to take personal inventory and admitting when we are wrong in the future

11. Seeking through prayer and meditation to improve your contact with God, according to your beliefs, asking only for knowledge of God's will and the power to carry it out

12. Carrying this message to other addicts and practicing these principles in all your affairs

What sets 12-step programs apart from other approaches is its emphasis on the spiritual dimension of recovery. Although the element of spirituality is not specific to a particular religion, some groups choose not to include it. Spirituality also involves a belief in or sense of connection to something greater than oneself, which is consistent with some of the newer models of psychotherapy.

Historically, 12-step treatment programs are linked largely to recovery from alcohol abuse and addiction. AA, the original 12-step program, has been supporting recovery since its inception in 1935. Over 1 million persons have achieved recovery through involvement in AA programs. At any one time, more than 100,000 men and women worldwide are involved in AA 12-step programs.

DID YOU KNOW?

Other Rehabilitation Programs

Although 12-step programs are very popular, there are a number of other programs that do not follow the 12-step guidelines. These include:

- Moderation Management, an alcohol education group for early-stage problem drinkers
- LifeRing, a secular abstinence support group
- Recovery, Inc., a skill-building group for dealing with emotional issues
- Secular Organizations for Sobriety, disease- and abstinence-based support groups
- Self-Management and Recovery Training (SMART) (formerly Rational Recovery), an alcohol, drug, and other addiction abstinence skills group
- Women for Sobriety, a disease- and abstinence-based support group with emphasis on self-empowerment

Addiction affects not only those recovering from drug abuse but also his or her family and friends. They, too, may need counseling. A number of support groups help them deal with the issues caused by alcohol or drug use. For example, Al-Anon helps families and friends of alcoholics. Alateen offers a similar recovery program for teens. Both programs are based on the 12 steps. The only requirement for membership in either group is having a relative or friend who is an alcoholic.

Issues in therapy

In treating drug abuse with psychotherapy, a number of issues complicate the process. One issue is the time and energy needed to overcome denial and get the client into treatment. In addition, the therapist must develop treatment goals early in the process and keep these goals at the forefront of treatment. Therapists must also develop a good rapport with the client and support him or her. An additional issue is that the therapist must stay abreast of the client's compliance with the overall treatment program, which may include monitoring attendance in different parts of the recovery program, providing regular urinalysis, and reporting use of any drugs. In the event of substitution therapy, such as methadone maintenance, it is important to record the different aspects of the treatment.

Family members can play an important role in recovery. Family and even close friends can facilitate the recovery process and help the teen create a better, more knowledgeable support network. Doing so may actually decrease the negative family behavior patterns that can slow recovery such as **codependence**, a set of compulsive behaviors that frequently develop between family members and a person within the family who has an addiction. Family programs can help participants improve communication and parenting skills. The National Institute on Drug Abuse claims that parents who take an active role in their children's lives by talking with them about drugs, monitoring their activities, getting to know their friends, and understanding their problems and personal concerns are more likely to raise teens who do not abuse drugs or alcohol.

The impact of peers (people of one's own age and social group) on treatment cannot be understated. Peers can provide a support network that encourages for rehabilitation and treatment. However, many of the peers in a teen's life may have actually contributed to the drug problem. Most recovery programs will work with teens in dealing appropriately with peer pressure, but often building new, more supportive peer networks will speed the recovery process.

Communication is critical to recovery, whether the communication is between the therapist and patient, family/friends and patient, or even from the patient to himself or herself. Many therapists encourage an internal dialog about one's own attitudes, actions, and behavior. Known as **self-talk**, this kind of communication can be important in overcoming psychological barriers to recovery.

Often self-talk is negative and demeaning. Some people have a tendency to be very hard on themselves, criticizing themselves for small failings or perceived weaknesses. Negative self-talk can lead to low self-esteem, which can hinder your ability to resist drugs as well as to recover from drug addiction. Positive self-talk is an important part of recovery because positive habits need to be reinforced. People learn not to be so hard on themselves when something does not go as planned, or when a potentially embarrassing event occurs. Substituting positive self-talk for negative self-talk is a good first step toward facing and dealing with your situation realistically.

Recovery can be a long-term process that often requires multiple attempts and many lifestyle changes. Several episodes of relapse (falling back into addiction) are not uncommon before achieving the long-term goal of being drug- or alcohol-free. In addition, there is little research that accurately measures success rates for different types of treatment and therapy. This means that finding the best treatment for a particular individual may be a long and difficult process. However, discovering the recovery plan that works best and sticking to it can be the first step in helping the addict once again gain control over his or her life.

See also: Dependence and Addiction; Drug Abuse, Causes of; Risk Factors and Risk Taking

FURTHER READING

Eisenberg, Arlene, Howard Eisenberg, and Al L. Mooney. *The Recovery Book.* New York: Workman Publishing Company, 1992.

Hawes, Gene and Anderson Hawes. *Addiction-Free: How to Help an Alcoholic or Addict Get Started on Recovery.* New York: Thomas Dunne Books, 2001.

Manville, Bill. *Cool, Hip, and Sober: 88 Ways to Beat Booze and Drugs.* New York: Forge Books, 2003.

■ RISK FACTORS AND RISK TAKING

Any behavior or set of circumstances that increase the chances of a person taking drugs. Having many risk factors for drug or alcohol abuse does not mean an individual will use drugs or alcohol. When all is said and done, a person still has choices.

The teen years are a time of change, growth, and exploration. New relationships and increased personal freedoms are among the challenges that involve both opportunities for personal growth and substantial risks. Teens need to be aware of the kinds of behavior that can increase the risk of using drugs. Knowing the risk factors can help teens avoid situations where drug use is likely to occur.

INDIVIDUAL AND PERSONAL FACTORS

Many factors tempt teens to engage in risk-taking behaviors. The desire for greater independence, individuality, and self-expression deepens as teens mature. They want greater control over their lives and their futures. While young teens (12- and 13-year-olds) depend heavily on adult supervisors, older teens (18- and 19-year-olds) are more independent and spend more time with peers (people one's own age and social group). Growing up takes time, but most teens are eager to move as quickly as possible.

The teen years are also a time of taking risks. Peers may encourage risk-taking behaviors such as speeding, skipping school, or experimenting with drugs. Peer pressure can have a strong influence on a teen's decision to engage in such behaviors.

However, every action has consequences. Teens who speed for thrills or to go along with their friends eventually find out the hard way how foolish and risky speeding is. Those who abuse drugs and alcohol learn the same hard lesson. What may have seemed a good idea the night before is regretted the day after. Understanding the consequences of risky behaviors in advance can be invaluable in making sound judgments and avoiding bad decisions.

To reduce exposure to the risk factors associated with drug and alcohol use follow a few basic rules:

- Don't hang out with people who use drugs and alcohol.
- Avoid going places or attending events where drugs and alcohol are consumed.
- Don't ride with anyone who has been drinking or using drugs.
- Before going to a party, make arrangements for a friend to act as a **designated driver**.

By understanding the consequences of actions in advance, teens might realize that what appears on the surface to be fun, exciting, and cool in actuality may be a giant hassle in the making.

FAMILY INFLUENCES

Families play a major role in the life of teens. Families with adult role models who abuse drugs or alcohol can have a negative influence on teens. Teens often imitate, or model, the behavior of authority figures, and a parent who uses drugs sets a bad example that teens might follow. According to the American Academy of Child and Adolescent Psychiatry, children raised in families with a history of drug or alcohol abuse are themselves at greater risk of abusing those substances. Additionally, families who use intimidation, violence, and abuse as parenting tools foster teens who run a much higher risk of using alcohol and drugs as coping mechanisms.

A positive family environment is one in which teens have support from adults to help them make a successful transition from childhood to adulthood. A positive family environment will also help both parents and teens weather tough times during that transition. Unfortunately, many teens do not feel supported by their family, especially when a request for advice results in ultimatums or threats. Having the support and understanding of one's family when making tough decisions can be priceless.

Establishing a situation of mutual respect within families is extremely helpful, but sometimes relationships like these are not possible. Identifying an adult outside the family circle who understands the difficulties a teen faces can be a helpful substitute when turning to family is not an option. Finding a special teacher, religious leader, counselor, or coach to discuss tough issues with can be most helpful, especially when support and perspective is needed.

Q & A

Question: Does moving around frequently increase the chances a teen will use drugs?

Answer: Moving frequently does not automatically mean that a teen will have problems with drugs. However, the more often a teen's family moves, the higher the risk of abusing substances. The reason? Teens who are uprooted frequently lack sufficient time to develop strong, trusting friendships. Sometimes teens in a new environment will unknowingly befriend teens who use drugs. Peer substance abuse is a strong indicator that a teen will also use drugs. For this reason, moving around can be a risk factor for substance abuse.

COMMUNITY INFLUENCES

Where a teen lives can be supportive or detrimental. The physical and socioeconomic situations that shape some communities increase the chances that local teens will become involved with drugs or alcohol. For example, communities located in run-down sections of town where the residents have little money or resources may have a greater likelihood of drug and alcohol use. Such communities often experience greater gang activity, which not only increases drug traffic but also the potential for violence. According to the 1997 National Youth Gang Survey, rural communities are not immune from drug and gang influences, but the number of gangs dealing drugs was greatest in and around big cities.

Economic factors definitely play a role in community drug and alcohol issues. According to the 1996 book *When Work Disappears: The World of the New Urban Poor*, when businesses move out of the inner city, residents are left with fewer legitimate opportunities to work and make a living. This, in turn, can lead to increased drug use in a community, especially in communities where unemployment is already high. Gangs typically establish or expand their drug business into lower socioeconomic areas within large metropolitan areas. The increased drug traffic and subsequent violence within these areas places a heavy burden on the teens living there. Drug use and the associated violence, elevated rates of HIV infection, and nonviolent crime such as prostitution are all-too-typical characteristics of living in poor areas.

Affluent communities also must deal with the influence of drugs and alcohol. Teens in wealthy suburbs often have large amounts of free time and cash to spend, which can lead them to experiment with drugs. Gangs realize the potential for sales to affluent youth and may service communities with drugs through local couriers. A recent example occurred in Plano, Texas, an upscale suburb of Dallas. In the late 1990s, Plano experienced a wave of **heroin** abuse that led to a number of overdoses among teens. A heroin-trafficking ring that targeted wealthy teens with lots of free time and money victimized Plano, named an "All-American City" in 1994. The police eventually arrested those responsible for trafficking heroin, but the episode left the community shaken. Plano parents had believed their community was safe from a drug that they associated with inner-city crime and violence.

Wealthier communities may take the position that drugs and drug dealers only happen in the "other" communities, and thus provide little support to teens. Conversely, less well-off communities may realize the need for teen support and establish services and centers to help teens in need. Regardless of whether it is rich or poor, every community chooses to be supportive of teens or not. Any community that believes it doesn't need to be concerned about drugs has a bigger problem than it can imagine.

Fact Or Fiction?

Cultural identification with friends of the same culture might reduce risk factors for drug abuse despite the influence of peer drug users, drug availability, or a parent's drug use.

Fact: The 1999 National Institute on Drug Abuse (NIDA) study "Ethnic Identification and Cultural Ties May Help Prevent Drug Use" found that cultural identification with friends of the same culture had a significant influence on teen drug use. An awareness of cultural history and tradition, identification with friends of the same culture, or participation in cultural activities can reduce the risk of drug use. Cultural influence can even be strong enough to offset the influence of peer drug users, drug availability, and a parent's drug use.

CULTURAL INFLUENCES

A wide variety of cultural factors, such as sexual preference or ethnic heritage, affect whether an individual will be vulnerable to alcohol and other drug use. Cultural influences can either significantly increase or substantially decrease the risk of teen drug and alcohol use. Cultural factors can also affect a teen's response to substance abuse treatment.

In some cultures, the use of certain drugs under tightly controlled situations is part of some religious rituals. For example, members of some Native American cultures take hallucinogenic drugs such as **peyote** as part of their religious ceremonies. However, the use of **illicit drugs** in cultural celebrations, rituals, or rites is the exception rather than the rule.

According to *Well Connected*, a health newsletter written and edited by medical faculty at Harvard University and Massachusetts General Hospital, alcoholism does vary among ethnic groups. Some, such as Irish and Native Americans, have a higher than average rate of alcoholism while others, such as Jewish and Asian Americans, have a lower risk. Some researchers feel these differences may represent cultural factors; others suggest that they reflect biological or genetic differences between different groups.

In 1999, NIDA published a research study titled "Ethnic Identification and Cultural Ties May Help Prevent Drug Use." The study found that ethnic identification may significantly influence drug use, and it identified important cultural issues that can impact drug use. For example, the study reported that Puerto Rican and African- American adolescents were less vulnerable to risk factors for drug use if they strongly identified with their communities and cultures. Members of the Asian community who responded to the study expressed the belief that drug abuse prevention programs can be more effective by including ethnic and cultural components into planning. For example, prevention programs should emphasize important cultural values that are at odds with or threatened by drug abuse. There is still some question about just how much impact cultural influences have in shaping antidrug behavior. However, in conjunction with family, personality, or positive peer influences, cultural factors may substantially reduce risk factors for drug abuse.

See also: Drugs and Criminal Activity; Drugs and Disease; Families, Communities, and Drug Abuse; Gangs and Drugs; Peer Pressure and Drugs

FURTHER READING
Monaghan, Lee F. *Bodybuilding, Drugs, and Risk.* New York: Routledge, 2001.

■ SCHOOL PERFORMANCE AND DRUG ABUSE

Relationship between academic and social performance in a school setting and drugs. Various studies have found that drug and alcohol use can have a negative impact on school attendance and performance. Drug use by peers and peer pressure are risk factors for teen drug abuse. Roughly 60 percent of high school teens report that drugs are used, kept, or sold at their schools. Students at these schools are three times more likely to smoke, drink, or use illegal drugs than students whose schools are substance-free.

ATTENDANCE AND ACADEMIC PERFORMANCE

A wide body of scientific literature shows a strong relationship between drug abuse and academic performance. According to the National Clearinghouse for Alcohol and Drug Information, teens that take drugs have a dropout rate five times greater than other students. Teens who abuse alcohol are four times more likely than other students to cut

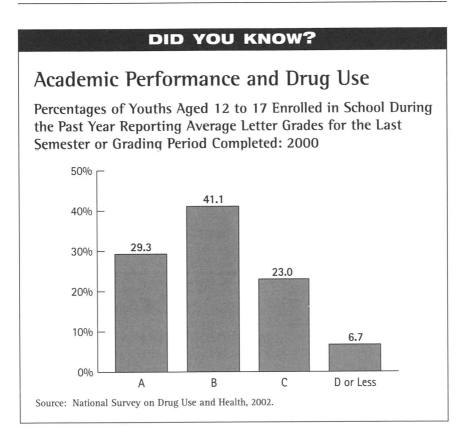

DID YOU KNOW?

Academic Performance and Drug Use

Percentages of Youths Aged 12 to 17 Enrolled in School During the Past Year Reporting Average Letter Grades for the Last Semester or Grading Period Completed: 2000

Source: National Survey on Drug Use and Health, 2002.

classes or skip school, and those who use **marijuana** are six times more likely to do so. These statistics are especially troubling because the majority of teens who later abuse drugs typically start their drug use with tobacco, alcohol, **inhalants**, and marijuana. These drugs are often called **gateway drugs** or entry-level substances because they are often the first substances in a progression of drug abuse.

For teens that stay in school, drug or alcohol use can result in academic failure. The 2000 National Survey on Drug Use and Health, a study sponsored by the Substance Abuse and Mental Health Services Administration (SAMHSA), found that alcohol, tobacco, and drug use produces an array of negative effects on academic performance. For example, only 6.7 percent of all teens ages 12–17 reported a letter grade of D or below for the previous semester, compared to 24.4 percent of teens who had used illegal drugs and 30 percent of those who used alcohol.

The survey also reported that the lower a teen's grade average, the more likely it is that he or she recently used cigarettes, alcohol, or an illicit drug. Only 6 percent of teens with an A average reported smoking cigarettes during the previous month, compared to 13 percent of those with a B average, 20 percent of those with a C average, and 36 percent of those with a D average or less.

In 2002, researchers at the University of Minnesota and the University of North Carolina at Chapel Hill conducted the National Longitudinal Study of Adolescent Health, the largest, most comprehensive survey of adolescents ever undertaken in the United States. Approximately 90,000 students in grades seven through 12 from 145 schools across the country participated. The purpose of the study was to identify factors that tend to protect teens from engaging in harmful behaviors such as alcohol and drug use.

The study found that repeating a grade seemed to increase the risk of substance abuse. Some 20 percent of teens are held back yearly, according to the study. Many teens view repeating a grade as proof of academic failure, which is a risk factor for drug and alcohol abuse. By contrast, academic success tends to reduce the chances that a teen will use drugs or alcohol.

Drug abuse not only takes an academic toll on students but also has a financial impact on schools. According to a recent study titled "Malignant Neglect: Substance Abuse and America's Schools" by the National Center on Addiction and Substance Abuse at Columbia University, the costs to schools associated with drugs include the costs associated with truancy, violence, property damage, lost productivity, teacher turnover, special education, school security, disciplinary programs, higher insurance costs, and legal expenses. The study estimated that these and related costs add 10 percent (approximately $41 billion) to the budgets of schools across the country, money that most schools are hard-pressed to find.

The study also detected a large gap between the way students and faculty members view drugs in relation to their school. Students and faculty were asked if they thought their school grounds were drug-free. While 89 percent of principals and 65 percent of teachers responded yes, only 34 percent of students claimed their schools were drug-free. In addition, only 5 percent of principals think students drink alcohol on school grounds, compared to 33 percent of students. One-half of all high school teachers think students who use marijuana every week can still do well in school, but only 23 percent of students think a user can navigate studies as well as a non-user.

TEENS SPEAK

I Have Witnessed the Impact of Drugs and Alcohol

I am a senior, and I have seen how many kids start out using cigarettes or alcohol thinking it's no big deal and then find themselves using much heavier drugs and ending up addicted. A lot of them drop out of school, but the ones who try to stick with it usually end up flunking out or are suspended for some drug- or violence-related issue. For the few drug users who remain, their grades are typically bad.

That is why I am really concerned that my little brother has started smoking and hanging around with a bad crowd. He is a smart kid, but he has low self-esteem. He is easily influenced by anyone who appears cool. Maybe he thinks less of himself because he is not as big and well-built as his athletic brothers, or maybe because he is the youngest in the family he feels he was treated differently. I really don't know why he doesn't believe in himself, all I know is that because he doesn't, he has a tendency to connect with some shady characters.

I am going to sit down and have a long talk with him about all this stuff. I am concerned though that he won't listen to me. I have considered talking with my health teacher about the issue. Ms. Simpson has my brother in class this year. I know he respects and likes her so I think he might listen to what she has to say. She will also keep track of him and make sure he is not heading in the wrong direction. He really is a good kid, but I know if he continues down this path he will end up like the others—out of school and without a good future.

SOCIAL ACTIVITIES AND DRUG USE

Drug and alcohol abuse also affects teen participation in extracurricular school activities such as athletics, cheerleading, academic competitions, or musical and artistic performances. The SAMHSA study found that participation in two or more activities was highest for teens with an A average and lowest for teens with a D or less than D average. Also, teens who participated in two or more activities during the previous year were less likely than those who participated in one activity or none to have used cigarettes, alcohol, or an illicit drug.

The study indicated that 16 percent of teens who took part in two or more activities during the previous year used alcohol, compared with 22 percent of those who did not participate at all or only took part in one activity. Similar results were found regarding illicit drug use and participation in teen activities. Teens who participated in one or fewer activities in the past year were twice as likely to have used an illicit drug compared with youths who participated in two or more youth activities.

However, simply participating in social or extracurricular activities does not protect a teen from exposure to drugs or alcohol. Some people believe that only certain social groups in school—often those who are shunned or considered misfits by a large percentage of students—abuse drugs and alcohol. The fact is, teen substance abuse can occur in any social group or school organization. For example, some school social clubs use alcohol and drugs as a part of their initiation ceremonies.

Often the initiation rites that social groups perform are nothing more than hazing—physical and psychological abuse that a prospective member of the group undergoes before being admitted. Hazing is an extreme form of peer pressure, in which the abuse is typically justified as a way to show one's loyalty to or solidarity with other members of the group. Alcohol and drugs can play a big part in hazing activities. A number of students in recent years have died as a result of alcohol poisoning or accidents caused by use of alcohol and drugs during hazing rituals.

No social group is immune to hazing activities. In the past, athletic clubs were most notorious for drug and alcohol abuse, but they are no longer alone. According to a 1999 study conducted by Alfred University, members of church groups, choir groups, marching bands, and cheerleading squads all report being hazed as new members. Hazing has become a major problem in American high schools and colleges. Almost half of students who belong to student groups reported being hazed. Given the fact that 91 percent of high school students belong to at least one group, you can see that hazing is a significant problem. However, it is just one symptom of the wider problem of drug and alcohol abuse in schools.

See also: Drug Abuse, Causes of; Peer Pressure and Drugs; Risk Factors and Risk Taking

■ SEXUAL BEHAVIOR AND DRUG ABUSE

Intimate contact with another person including but not limited to sexual intercourse. The use of drugs and alcohol affects sexual behavior, because drugs reduce inhibitions and cloud judgment, making teens more vulnerable to faulty decision making. In its 2002 Youth Risk Behavior Surveillance System (YRBSS), the Centers for Disease Control and Prevention (CDC) reported that approximately 33 percent of U.S. teens are sexually active and roughly 7 percent had sex before the age of 13. About 25 percent of sexually active teens have used drugs and/or alcohol while engaging in sexual intercourse.

Not only do alcohol and drugs cloud the decision about whether to engage in sex, but they also may affect the decision to use protection. The CDC YRBSS points out that only 60 percent of those teens who recently engaged in sexual intercourse reported using a condom, which means that nearly one-half of all teens are at risk of **sexually transmitted diseases** (STDs).

Fact Or Fiction?

Drug and alcohol use is associated with increased STD transmission.

Fact: Research has found a relationship between alcohol and other drug use and high-risk sexual behavior among heterosexuals. A teen's high-risk sexual behavior and problem-drinking patterns were strongly predictive of self-reported sexually transmitted disease.

Decisions about whether to use a condom may be influenced by drug and alcohol abuse. Teens who abuse drugs or alcohol tend to engage in more risk-taking behaviors because those substances reduce inhibitions and impair judgment and reasoning skills. The result may be a failure to consider or dismiss the importance of wearing a condom. Considering the value of condoms in preventing sexually transmitted diseases such as HIV (the virus that causes AIDS), teens cannot afford to risk a failure of judgment in such a situation.

Q & A

Question: What are "beer goggles?"

Answer: The phrase "beer goggles" describes the influence that alcohol and drugs have on one's perception of another person's appearance. Guys often use this term in a demeaning fashion. However, the term is not connected to a specific gender. Males and females equally can fall prey to the impact of drugs and alcohol on their judgment and decision-making ability. Research sponsored by the National Institute on Drug Abuse and the National Institute on Alcohol Abuse and Alcoholism has shown that drug and alcohol use can negatively affect a teen's judgment about sexual (and other) behaviors, increasing the chance that users will engage in unplanned and unprotected sex. This activity can place teens at increased risk for contracting HIV and other STDs from infected sex partners.

DATE RAPE DRUGS

Recently the media has focused attention on **date rape drugs**, substances that are used to render a person unconscious and susceptible to rape. These drugs, which are typically slipped into a drink, leave the victim with no recollection of what happened. Date rape drugs generally fall under the heading of **depressants**, because they depress the functions of the central nervous system, causing symptoms such as drowsiness, dizziness, nausea, visual disturbances, and a sense of **euphoria** (feeling of extreme elation and well-being). Three substances are commonly identified as date rape drugs: Rohypnol, GHB (gamma-hydroxybutyrate), and ketamine. Two other less popular chemical depressants related to GHB are GBL (gamma-butyrolactone), and 1,4 butanediol, sometimes called BD.

Rohypnol, which may be the most widely used date rape drug, is actually a potent **tranquilizer** that was developed for use as a surgical anesthetic (painkiller), muscle relaxant, or sleeping pill. It is the trade name for the drug flunitrazepam, a benzodiazepine. On the street, Rohypnol has a wide array of names, including roofies, rope, ruffies, ruffles, Roche, forget-me pill, Roffies, rophies, R-2s, LaRocha, Mexican Valium, rib, roach, and roofenol.

The effects of Rohypnol include muscle relaxation and a slowing of motor (muscular) response. It also decreases blood pressure, causes urinary retention, and produces an alcohol-like intoxication. The most profound effect of the drug is that it produces anterograde amnesia—the inability to remember events that take place after the drug was taken. It is this aspect of the drug that causes it to be so widely used as a date rape drug. The effects of Rohypnol kick in roughly 10–20 minutes after ingestion and last from two to eight hours. When Rohypnol is mixed with alcohol, it results in lack of inhibition along with the amnesia. The effects can last from eight to 24 hours.

Rohypnol is odorless and tasteless. However, due to its unintended use as a date rape drug, the company changed the formula so a color appears when Rohypnol is dissolved in liquid. In the past, Rohypnol was undetectable in drinks. The reformulated pills now take 45 minutes to dissolve, leave a chalky film, and turn a light-colored drink blue. It may take some time to remove all the old formula off the streets, so teens need to be vigilant.

Rohypnol is available in three different forms: as a .5-milligram oblong tablet, a 1.0-milligram tablet, and a 1.0-milligram per liter injectable solution.

If someone shows signs of being drunk—dizziness, confusion, or other sudden unexplained symptoms—after drinking any beverage, chances are he or she has been drugged. If you suspect that you or someone you know has been drugged, seek medical attention immediately. Rohypnol by itself is rarely life threatening, but when mixed with alcohol it can slow certain vital functions—such as heartbeat and breathing—to dangerously low levels. Victims are at risk of coma or even death from respiratory failure.

Gamma-hydroxybutyrate, or GHB, goes by a variety of street names, including liquid ecstasy, liquid X, easy lay, grievous bodily harm, saltwater, scoop, and Gamma-O. It is an odorless, colorless, liquid depressant that acts like an anesthetic. GHB acquired its reputation as a date rape drug because of the tranquility, sensuality, and loss of inhibitions it produces, particularly in women. GHB also promotes hormones that stimulate muscle growth. Bodybuilders used to take GHB, but its use has been banned since 1990 because of its side effects. At lower doses, GHB produces euphoria similar to alcohol, generating the feeling of being relaxed, happy, and sociable. At higher doses, dizziness, vomiting, and muscle spasms are possible. GHB produces symptoms of lethargy, extreme intoxication, impaired judgment, nausea, vomiting, and dizziness. It can also cause unconsciousness, **depression**, seizures, severe respiratory depression, and coma. Once the drug is consumed, symptoms appear within 15–20 minutes and can last two to three hours. However some effects may continue to linger for an entire day. The symptoms are more dangerous when GHB is slipped into alcohol, because both drugs depress central nervous system functioning. Symptoms such as respiratory depression and coma are a result of mixing alcohol and GHB. The combination has caused a number of deaths.

One of the most dangerous aspects of GHB use is the unpredictability of dosages. Because GHB is manufactured in basements, the strength and size of a dose are inconsistent, making it unpredictable and especially dangerous. A dose that produced no serious problems one time may result in an overdose the next time. Also, a variety of factors can impact dosage including body weight and the amount of food an individual has consumed. There is no "safe" dose of GHB, and previous experience with the drug is not necessarily a reliable predictor of future experiences.

Although GHB is produced primarily in liquid form, it can also be found in powder or capsule form. GHB is colorless, odorless, and has a slightly salty taste that makes it easy to mistake for a highly carbonated health drink. It dissolves easily in liquids and can be added to bottled water or hidden in other containers. The fact that it can be easily added to a drink without the victim's knowledge increases the dangers associated with the drug.

Ketamine is a relatively new date rape drug. It is a legal drug that is used as an animal tranquilizer due to its anesthetic characteristics. Ketamine has a wide array of street names, which include K, Special K, vitamin K, and Ket. Its effects have been compared to those of **PCP** and include **hallucinations**, amnesia, and dissociation—a feeling that the mind is separated from the body. Ketamine can also produce near-death experiences, depression, long-term memory and cognitive difficulties, and fatal respiratory problems. Ketamine is typically a liquid that is injected, applied to smokable material, or consumed in drinks. It can also be found as a powder or pill.

HIV AND DRUG ABUSE

In 1981 when **HIV** (the virus that causes AIDS) was recognized, unprotected sexual intercourse and the sharing of **intravenous drug** needles were identified as the two primary methods of transmission. Since those early days, much new information has been discovered about HIV. One of those discoveries identified the increased risk of infection from anabolic steroid injections. Since steroids are injected into the muscles, not the veins, the name intravenous drug use has changed to **injection drug** use to include steroid abuse. One fact that remains constant—sharing drug needles increases the risk of HIV/AIDs.

Teen use of injection drugs nationally is minimal; less than 2 percent of teens responding to the 2003 National Institute on Drug Abuse "Monitoring the Future" study reported using **heroin**, the most widely abused injection drug. However, for those who do inject drugs and share needles, the risk of HIV is ever present. Sharing needles with anyone is highly risky behavior.

A person can be infected with HIV and not show outward symptoms for years. In the meantime he or she transmits the virus to other people. The same scenario applies to unprotected sexual intercourse. Unless a blood test is performed, it's almost impossible to know someone's HIV status. So the rule is, always assume someone is infected and make decisions accordingly. According to the National Center on Health Statistics, AIDS killed more than 14,000 Americans in 2001. Teens need to protect themselves and the best way to do that is prevention.

SEXUAL AND REPRODUCTIVE FUNCTION

Ironically, some of the drugs that increase a teen's risk of engaging in sexual activity can also impair his or her sexual and reproductive functioning. A large number of studies have shown a link between alcohol use and sexual dysfunction. According to "Medications That May Contribute to Sexual Disorders," a 1997 article in the *Journal of Family Practice*, chronic alcohol abuse can suppress normal hormonal functions such as sexual arousal. It can also reduce the size of the testes. The 2003 Health Professionals Follow-up Study reported that impotence was more common among men who drank alcohol.

Drugs other than alcohol can also have a negative effect on sexual function. The 1997 article reported that **cocaine** use may hinder the ability to attain an erection or achieve orgasm. Like cocaine, chronic use of **amphetamines** also affects orgasm and erection. **Barbiturates** can impact sexual function as well by reducing desire and making it difficult to achieve erection or orgasm. A 1996 article, "Sexual Side Effects of Antidepressants," that appeared in the *Journal of Sex and*

Marital Therapy, found that **antidepressant** medications may also reduce sexual desire and interfere with orgasm. The wide range of sexual problems associated with drug use undermines the myth that using drugs enhances pleasure or is somehow "sexy."

See also: Drugs and Disease; Drugs and Drinking; Injection Drugs; Risk Factors and Risk Taking

FURTHER READING
Plant, Moira and Martin A. Plant. *Risk Takers: Alcohol, Drugs, Sex, and Youth.* New York: Routledge, 1992.

■ STEROIDS, ANABOLIC
Artificially manufactured drugs derived from the male sex hormone testosterone. Athletes have long used steroids to develop greater muscle mass and strength despite dangerous effects. In recent years, anabolic steroids have become popular among teens, especially teen athletes. What was thought to be a problem only among college and professional athletes has now become a concern in middle schools and high schools across the nation.

MEDICAL USE
Unlike many other abused drugs, steroids have medicinal value. The steroids used most frequently in medicine are cortisone and various synthetic offshoots of cortisone. These drugs are used for a variety of skin ailments, rheumatoid arthritis, asthma, allergies, and various eye diseases. Steroids can also be used to treat a malfunctioning adrenal cortex, the part of the brain that regulates the body's response to stress. They have also been found to help treat delayed puberty, some types of impotence, and wasting of the body caused by HIV infection. (HIV is the virus that causes AIDS.)

ILLEGAL USE AND SIDE EFFECTS
Concern about steroid abuse grew after scientists discovered serious side effects with the drugs' use. In 1974, this new information, along with a newly developed method of testing athletes, led the International Olympics Committee to ban the use of steroids.

TEENS SPEAK

I'm Built Like a Bean Pole

I have never been that good in school, and my body is not what you would call developed. So I basically didn't fit in with any group. But I recently got interested in lifting weights with a couple of my buddies. All of a sudden I feel better about myself and my confidence is the best it's ever been. We are really committed to lifting, never missing a day. I can see the difference in my body even after only a few weeks of training. I know it will take time and effort but I am willing to pay the price.

Not long after we began training, one of my lifting buddies showed up with a pill that he says will help us get bigger and stronger faster. The pill is a steroid, and he told us it is harmless and said if we really want to get really big we can "stack" steroids. I wasn't totally sure about this, so I went to talk with Coach Smith. She told me that "stacking" is when two or more anabolic steroids are taken together. People who stack mix oral and injection steroids and sometimes add drugs like stimulants or painkillers. She said the idea behind stacking is an unproven belief that the different drugs interact to produce a greater effect on muscle size. She also said we needed to be careful because steroid use had some really nasty side effects. It can cause acne, reduce a guy's sperm count, shrink the testicles, lead to impotence, result in difficulty or pain in urinating, baldness, and *even* irreversible breast enlargement. She said that the long-term effects can include cancer and possibly heart attacks and strokes.

After hearing the facts and doing some soul-searching, I told my buddies they can do what they want, but I want to do this on my own—not the cheater's way by using steroids. I may not get as big as fast but I will have done it on my own. That makes me feel good.

Despite the ban, steroid abuse continues to be a problem in international sports. Athletes are regularly accused of using performance-enhancing steroids at not only the Olympic Games but also other athletic competitions. In the 1998 Los Angeles Olympics, 100-meter dash champion Ben Johnson was disqualified after he failed a test for steroids. In 2004, the United States government launched an investigation into steroid use in major league baseball.

With the enormous salaries paid to many professional athletes, some seem to think the benefits of steroid use may be worth the risk. It is not. While athletes who use steroids gain an unfair advantage in competitions, the advantage comes at a high price. Steroids have been shown to produce serious psychological and physiological side effects, including increased aggressive behavior and cancer of the liver. The National Institute on Drug Abuse (NIDA) points out that in male teens, anabolic steroid abuse can reduce sperm production, shrink the testicles, and cause impotence and irreversible breast enlargement. In female teens, the development of secondary masculine characteristics such as deepening of the voice and excessive body hair may occur. Anabolic steroids may also stunt bone growth and cause permanent damage to the heart, liver, and kidneys.

Those who inject anabolic steroids and share the needles increase their chances of developing HIV and other blood-borne infections. The practice of shooting up steroids actually caused health officials worldwide to change the name of a key mode of transmission for HIV and AIDS. Because steroids are injected into the muscle—and not intravenously, as many illegal drugs are—the designation **intravenous drug** use was changed to injection drug use to include the risk of HIV from the sharing of steroid needles.

The threat to teens from anabolic steroid abuse is real and growing. NIDA has been collecting information about the use of the drug among students for 25 years. Its 1999 "Monitoring the Future" study showed an increase in anabolic steroid use among eighth and 10th graders. The survey discovered that roughly 3 percent of eighth, 10th, and 12th graders had taken anabolic steroids at least once in their lives. These statistics show a significant increase from the 1991 survey, which was the first year data on steroid abuse was collected.

A comparison of the 1991 and 1999 studies also showed that fewer 12th graders in 1999 believed that taking steroids is risky behavior. The decline is a particularly troubling development, because perceived risk indicates how seriously teens regard the threat posed by a particular substance. A decline in the perceived risk of a substance is typically followed by an increase in its use.

SOCIAL ISSUES

American society places a high regard on body image and many teens will spend large sums of money and take drastic measures to improve their physical appearance. This obsession has increased substantially the number of teens battling eating disorders and having plastic surgeries and breast augmentations. In 1997 the Centers for Disease Control and Prevention reported that the eating disorder anorexia nervosa was the third most common chronic illness in adolescent women. Victims of anorexia are dangerously thin and obsessively concerned about their weight. About 90 percent of reported cases of eating disorders are in females, but the rate for males seems to be increasing. However, males who have concerns about body image typically want to build up their muscles and are thus more likely to abuse steroids. Although some females use steroids, their use is more common among males.

As the science behind muscular development and performance enhancement evolves, researchers are introducing new techniques that provide athletes with opportunities to reach optimum performance without steroids. The truth is, it takes hard work to achieve optimum performance no matter what method is used. Those who wish to do so should consider taking the following steps:

- Decide on a realistic goal.
- Research nutritional plans and workout schedules to fit that goal and your time schedule.
- Include time for mental and spiritual development. A stress management course or a mental imagery program may also be valuable.
- Plan your time; develop a reasonable schedule, especially in the beginning, when new habits need to be developed and old ones broken.
- Work your plan. Do not let yourself be sidetracked. The beginning is always the toughest. Sticking with any plan requires discipline and self-control.
- Establish a fitting reward; rewards that can be earned on a weekly or monthly basis are great motivators in addition to a big reward when the overall goal is achieved.

It matters little if the goal is trying to reach the Olympics or just to get in better physical shape. To accomplish each step in a plan requires dedication, self-discipline, and motivation. Many athletes find it helpful to train with a partner. Having someone to keep you on track on a day when your motivation is low is valuable. A partner also makes following the plan more fun.

See also: Drugs and Disease; Injection Drugs; Media Messages and Counteradvertising Campaigns

■ SUICIDE AND DRUGS
See: Depression and Drugs; Drugs and Drinking; Morbidity and Mortality

■ SYNTHETIC DRUGS
See: Club and Designer Drugs

■ TREATMENT PROGRAMS
See: Rehabilitation and Treatment

■ WITHDRAWAL
See: Rehabilitation and Treatment

■ WORKPLACE DRUG ABUSE
Use of illegal drugs while on the job. Drug abuse in the workplace is a real problem in the United States. For example, coworkers may have to work harder to pick up the slack for workers who are using drugs. Absenteeism may rise, requiring employers to add staff to cover for absent employees. Also, those who take drug utilize health benefits more frequently than other employees, raising insurance rates for everyone. In addition, roughly half of all workplace accidents are drug-related. Because of higher turnover rates among drug abusers, employers find themselves having to assume the additional cost of replacing workers more often. As these costs mount, company profits decline.

Teens often underplay the seriousness of using drugs or alcohol on the job. However, even a simple task like climbing a ladder can result in serious injury if someone trips because he or she is "high." The chances of getting hurt increase substantially when attempting more dangerous tasks such as operating power equipment. Even if a workplace accident is not life threatening, it can create significant hardships. Breaking an arm or leg on the job because of an accident caused by being high on drugs or alcohol can ruin a summer or force someone to drop out of athletics or other activities.

INCIDENCE AND COST OF WORKPLACE SUBSTANCE ABUSE

According to the 1997 National Household Survey on Drug Abuse, 7.7 percent of all American workers surveyed admitted to using alcohol or drugs at the workplace. About 9 percent of employees in small businesses (those employing fewer than 25 people) reported taking drugs at work, compared to 8 percent in medium-sized businesses (25–499 employees) and 5.8 percent in large businesses (500 or more employees). Some 70 percent of all illicit drug users were employed full-time, a total of over 6 million people. About one-quarter of these individuals both used drugs and drank heavily.

Alcohol, **marijuana** (an illicit drug that alters mood and distorts the way the user experiences sight, sound, or other senses), and **cocaine** (an illicit drug that increases energy and alertness and elevates confidence) are the drugs most frequently abused in the workplace and therefore cause the greatest problems. According to the Department of Health and Human Services' Substance Abuse and Mental Health Services Administration, alcoholics and problem drinkers are four to eight times more likely to be absent from work, and substance abusers average five missed days of work per month. Substance abusers are also 33 percent less productive than sober workers. The average substance abuser costs his or her employer $7,000 in lost productivity each year. In 1995, productivity losses attributed to alcohol alone reached $119 billion.

Workplace accidents are far more common among drug and alcohol abusers than among other workers. Workplace drug abusers are 3.6 times more likely to suffer a work-related injury and five times more likely to file a worker's compensation claim. Between 38 and 50 percent of all worker's compensation claims are related to drug or alcohol abuse. Forty percent of fatal industrial accidents involve alcohol abuse.

In 1986 the Hazelden Foundation, which provides counseling and treatment for substance abuse, issued a report that identified the occupations with the heaviest drinking and highest rate of illicit drug use. Topping the list were food preparation workers, waiters, waitresses, and bartenders at 19 percent, construction workers at 14 percent, service occupations at 13 percent, and transportation and material moving workers at 10 percent.

Less noticeable risks of drug and alcohol abuse also can have an impact on a company's productivity and profitability. Such risks include low morale, increased absenteeism among nonabusers, and high illness rates. These conditions often arise when an employer is aware of drug or alcohol abuse by an employee but does nothing to address the problem. Employees who do not abuse drugs or alcohol begin to question whether the employer values hard work and dedication in his or her employees.

The reality of the problem was brought home in a 1998 article, "New Perspectives for Worksite Alcohol Strategies: Results from a Corporate Drinking Study." The study revealed that roughly 20 percent of American workers claimed that they needed to work harder or redo work because of work done incorrectly by a colleague who abused drugs. They also reported covering for a coworker's poor performance due to substance abuse or being exposed to danger or injury as a result of a fellow employee's drinking.

DRUG-FREE WORKPLACES

The Drug-Free Workplace Act of 1988 requires that all businesses receiving federal funds provide a drug-free workplace. Under the law employers are required to:

- Inform employees in writing that making, buying, selling, possessing, or using illegal drugs is prohibited in the workplace. The statement should also state the actions that will be taken against employees who violate the policy.

- Establish a program to make employees aware of the dangers of drug abuse in the workplace, the policy of maintaining a drug-free workplace, available drug counseling, rehabilitation, and employee assistance programs, and penalties for drug abuse violations.

- Notify employees that they must abide by the terms of the policy statement and let their employer know within five days if they have been convicted of a drug violation in the workplace.

- Notify the federal government that an employee has been convicted of a criminal drug violation in the workplace within 10 days of receiving notice of the violation.

■ Penalize the employee or require him or her to participate in a drug abuse assistance or rehabilitation program.

■ Make an ongoing, good-faith effort to maintain a drug-free workplace by meeting the requirements of the act.

To ensure a drug-free workplace, many employers have instituted preemployment drug testing, as well as routine spot testing for drug use among current employees. American companies spent an estimated $1 billion in 1998 on drug testing. A 2000 study by the American Management Association found that 78.5 percent of

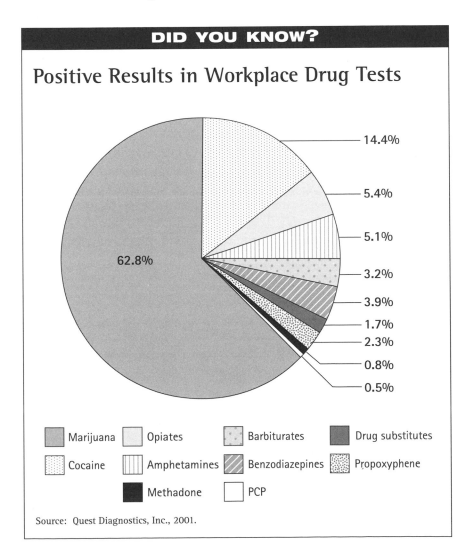

DID YOU KNOW?

Positive Results in Workplace Drug Tests

14.4%
5.4%
5.1%
3.2%
3.9%
1.7%
2.3%
0.8%
0.5%

62.8%

Marijuana   Opiates   Barbiturates   Drug substitutes

Cocaine   Amphetamines   Benzodiazepines   Propoxyphene

Methadone   PCP

Source: Quest Diagnostics, Inc., 2001.

manufacturing firms tested new hires for drug use, and 42.2 percent tested all of their employees. Other industries that tested over one-half of new hires for drug use included wholesale and retail (63 percent) and general services (60.3 percent). By contrast, financial services companies tested only 35.8 percent of new hires and just 18.8 percent of current employees. The figures for business and professional services firms were similar: 36 percent test new hires, while only 18.4 percent test current employees.

Preemployment drug testing is not the only way companies try to lower rates of drug and alcohol abuse among their employees. Other methods include providing employees with information about the dangers of drugs and alcohol abuse, following written policies on abuse to the letter, and offering assistance to employees who have addictions. Although these actions may seem minor, they can have a considerable impact on workplace drug use.

Drug testing laws are constantly changing. Because of changes in regulations, employers and employees alike need to continually monitor these laws. The federal laws that impact drug testing include the National Labor Relations Act, Title VII, and the Americans with Disabilities Act. Among the other laws that deal with workplace drug use are the Family and Medical Leave Act, workers' compensation statutes, unemployment compensation statutes, and federal privacy laws. State guidelines also need to be considered. With all these laws involved, it's easy to see why drug testing is so complicated.

See also: Law on Drugs, The; Morbidity and Mortality; Risk Factors and Risk Taking

HOTLINES AND HELP SITES

Alateen

URL: http://www.al-anonalateen.org

Phone: 1-888-AL-ANON (8 A.M.–6 P.M. ET, Mon.–Fri.)

Affiliation: Part of Al-Anon, an organization of relatives and friends of alcoholics

Mission: To help young people deal with problems of alcohol in their families or among friends

Program: Provides regular meetings of young people to discuss their problems and help each other to face them

Alcohol Treatment Referral Hotline

Phone: 1-800-ALCOHOL (24 hours a day, 7 days a week)

The CDC National AIDS Hotline

Phone: 1-800-342-AIDS; 1-800-344-SIDA (Spanish); 1-800-AIDS-TTY (TDD) (24 hours a day, 7 days a week)

Affiliation: Centers for Disease Control and Prevention, an agency of the federal government

Program: Trained specialists offer anonymous, confidential HIV/AIDS information, answer questions about HIV/AIDS, and provide referrals to appropriate services and service agencies throughout the United States

Center for Substance Abuse Treatment

URL: http://csat.samhsa.gov

Phone: 1-800-662-HELP (24 hours a day, 7 days a week)

Affiliation: U.S. Department of Health and Human Services

Mission: To develop and promote better treatment for substance abuse

Cocaine Anonymous
URL: http://www.ca.org
Mission: To help cocaine users break their addiction through mutual help and support
Program: 12-step treatment program for cocaine addiction

Cocaine Hotline
Phone: 1-800-COCAINE (24 hours a day, 7 days a week)

CyberSober
URL: http://www.cybersober.com
Mission: To provide the most comprehensive recovery and prevention resource on the Internet
Program: Provides online support for 12-step support groups, including schedules, maps, and driving directions for local support group meetings across the United States

Freevibe
URL: http://freevibe.com
Affiliation: National Youth Anti-Drug Media Campaign
Mission: To provide information to young people about alcohol and drugs and help kids find alternative interests and activities

Intervention Center
URL: http://www.intervention.com
Phone: 1-800-422-3213
Mission: To assist family and friends in confronting addicts and persuading them to break their addictions
Program: Provides interventional resources for alcoholism, drug addiction, gambling, computer addiction, and other self-destructive behavior

Marijuana Anonymous
URL: http://www.marijuana-anonymous.org
Phone: 1-800-766-6779
Mission: To help marijuana users break their addiction through mutual help and support
Program: 12-step program for treating marijuana addiction

National Council on Alcoholism and Drug Dependence
URL: http://www.ncadd.org
Phone: 1-800-NCA-CALL (24 hours a day, 7 days a week)
Program: Provides public education and information about alcohol and drug abuse, treatment, and recovery

Nar-Anon
URL: http://www.naranon.com
Phone: 1-800-477-6291 (24 hours a day, 7 days a week)
Mission: To help relatives and friends of addicts recover from the effects of living with an addict
Program: 12-step program for relatives and friends of drug addicts

Narcotics Anonymous World Services
URL: http://www.na.org
Phone: 1-818-773-9999
Program: 12-step program for treating drug addiction

Sober Recovery
URL: http://www.soberrecovery.com
Mission: To provide resources for those seeking help from alcoholism, addiction, and mental health issues
Program: Offers an online list of rehabilitation and treatment centers, sober living houses, recovery-related Web sites, and referrals and information for treatment programs for adults or adolescents

GLOSSARY

abstinence the practice of refraining from a behavior, especially risky behavior such as alcohol, tobacco, or drug use

accidental overdose a dangerously large dose of a drug taken by mistake

AIDS (acquired immune deficiency syndrome) medical condition in which the body's immune system is so weakened that even mild infections can cause serious illness or death

amphetamines synthetically produced stimulants that improve alertness, reduce fatigue, and elevate mood

antianxiety drugs prescription drugs used to reduce anxiety and nervousness

antidepressants prescription drugs that prevent or relieve depression

barbiturates prescription drugs that depress the central nervous system; used to treat anxiety, tension, and sleep disorders

bipolar disorder a brain disorder that causes unusual shifts in a person's mood, energy, and ability to function; also known as manic-depressive illness

central nervous system the part of the nervous system consisting of the brain and spinal cord

cocaine illicit drug, derived from the coca plant, that increases energy and alertness and elevates self-confidence

codependence condition in which a person close to a substance abuser behaves in ways that unconsciously support the user's habit

date rape drug drug administered without the user's consent that causes unconsciousness and makes the victim helpless against sexual assault

delinquency cases crimes in which a juvenile is treated as an adult under the law

delusions persistent beliefs that have no basis in reality

depressants drugs, including alcohol, tranquilizers, and inhalants, that slow the functioning of the central nervous system, causing relaxation, drowsiness, and loss of motor control

designated driver a person who remains sober to provide safe transportation for people who are drinking or using drugs

designer drugs synthetically produced illicit substances that produce a wide range of drug effects; also called club drugs

detoxification the process of gradually removing a drug from an addict's system

drug psychosis a loss of touch with reality produced by an adverse drug reaction

euphoria a feeling of extreme elation and well-being

felony a serious crime, such as murder or arson, punishable by one year or more in a state or federal prison

forfeiture the seizure of assets believed to have been acquired through the trafficking or sale of drugs

gateway drugs substances whose use is believed to lead to the abuse of other drugs; alcohol, tobacco, and marijuana are considered the main gateway drugs

hallucinations false or distorted perceptions caused by the use of some drugs

hallucinogens illicit drugs whose main effect is to produce hallucinations

hepatitis an infectious disease that can cause serious liver damage; often spread through sharing of injection drug equipment

heroin illicit drug derived from the Asian poppy that causes drowsiness, relieves pain, and produces euphoria

HIV (human immunodeficiency virus) virus that attacks the body's immune system and causes AIDS (acquired immune deficiency syndrome); frequently spread through sharing of injection drug equipment

intentional overdose a dangerously large dose of a drug taken deliberately, typically as a means of committing suicide

intravenous drugs drugs administered by injection into a vein

juvenile legal term for a person under the age of consent; in most states, a person under 18 years of age

legally drunk having a blood alcohol concentration of 0.10 grams of alcohol per deciliter of blood

LSD (lysergic acid diethalymide) widely used synthetic hallucinogen; also known as acid

marijuana illicit drug derived from the plant *Cannabis sativa* that produces relaxation, alters mood, and distorts the way the user experiences sight, sound, or other senses

mental illness medical disorder that can cause distressful effects ranging from mild sleep problems or relationship troubles to drug addiction or suicide

mescaline a mind-altering drug in the form of a white, crystalline powder

methamphetamines family of illicit nervous system stimulants that are related to amphetamines and which have similar but much more intense effects

opiates family of drugs derived from the Asian poppy that includes opium, morphine, and heroin

paranoia extreme and unreasonable feelings of persecution

PCP (phencyclidine) powerful illicit central nervous system depressant originally used as an anesthetic; also known as angel dust

physical dependence dependence on a substance for normal physical or psychological functioning

prescription drug drug whose use is legal only when prescribed by a medical professional

psychological dependence intense craving for a drug that is not accompanied by physical dependence

psychosis a mental disorder characterized by loss of touch with reality

schizophrenia a mental disorder that causes a separation between the thought processes and the emotions

sedative drug used to induce sleep or unconsciousness

self-talk the things one says to oneself about one's own competence, skills, and self-image

sexually active currently participating in sexual behavior

sexually transmitted diseases (STDs) diseases transmitted widely or primarily by sexual contact

social skills ability to make friends, deal successfully with other people, and set appropriate limits on your own behavior

stimulant drug, such as caffeine, nicotine, amphetamines, or cocaine, that tends to elevate mood, and increase alertness and energy

street sales sales of small amounts of illicit drugs to individual users

tolerance the need to use larger doses of a substance to produce the desired effect

trafficking the transport and sale of large amounts of illicit drugs to drug dealers

tranquilizer drug intended to make the user calm or incapable of physical resistance

trigger the act of setting off or initiating

withdrawal a condition caused by stopping the use of a drug and marked by adverse physical reactions such as nausea, sweating, and convulsions

INDEX

Page numbers in **bold** indicate extensive coverage of a topic. Page numbers in *italic* indicate graphs or sidebars.